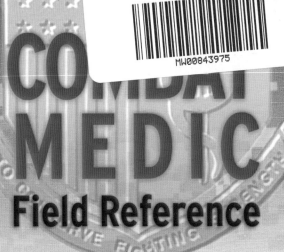

COMBAT MEDIC
Field Reference

Editor
Casey Bond, MPAS, PA-C

Contributing Editors
SFC Teroder Hudson, 91W
SSG Nadine Kahla, 91W
SSG Curtis Mitchell, 91W
SSG (P) Jeffrey Sliva, 91W
Donald L. Parsons, MPAS, PA-C
Meredith J. Hansen, MPH, PA-C

Warrior Ethos

I will always place the mission first.
I will never accept defeat.
I will never quit.
I will never leave a fallen comrade.

JONES AND BARTLETT PUBLISHERS
Sudbury, Massachusetts
BOSTON   TORONTO   LONDON   SINGAPORE

Jones and Bartlett Publishers

World Headquarters
Jones and Bartlett Publishers
40 Tall Pine Drive
Sudbury, MA 01776
978-443-5000
info@jbpub.com
www.jbpub.com

Jones and Bartlett Publishers International
Barb House, Barb Mews
London W6 7PA
United Kingdom

Jones and Bartlett Publishers Canada
6339 Ormindale Way
Mississauga, ON L5V 1J2
Canada

ISBN-13: 978-0-7637-3563-0
ISBN-10: 0-7637-3563-9

Production Credits
Chief Executive Officer: Clayton Jones
Chief Operating Officer: Donald W. Jones, Jr.
Publisher, Public Safety: Kim Brophy
Manufacturing Buyer: Therese Connell
Production Editor: Susan Schultz
Text and Cover Design: Anne Spencer
Composition: Shepherd Incorporated
Cover Photograph: © Laura Rauch/AP Photo
Printing and Binding: Transcontinental Metrolitho

Writing in the field reference
For making permanent notes, use a felt-tip pen such as a Sharpie™ and allow the ink to dry thoroughly (may take as long as 30 minutes). For temporary notes, erase as soon as possible (within 10 minutes preferably) with alcohol.

6048

Printed in Canada

10 09 08 07   10 9 8 7 6 5 4

Contents

Preface

The word for "healer" in ancient Greek is *iatros* meaning "remover of arrows."

The ability to save lives in war, conflicts, and humanitarian interventions is multi-factorial. Throughout time the Combat Medic has been a major contributor to this mission. The first medical care above the level of first aid is the task of the Combat Medic.

Today's Combat Medic must be an expert in emergency medical care, force health protection, limited primary care, evacuation, and Warrior Skills.

Combat Medic training has changed in the past decade. Lessons learned in previous conflicts and requirements for Army transformation have been incorporated into training. The Combat Medic of today is the most technically advanced conventional medic ever produced by the United States Army. The depth of understanding of anatomy and physiology and the sophistication of the skills the Combat Medic must master requires an intense dedication to the mission-craft of the Combat Medic.

This field-craft handbook is in recognition of the special needs of the Combat Medic.

The Combat Medic encompasses the best of the Army Medical Department. Whether required to work in austere environments or on a hospital ward these Soldiers have proven to be invaluable to Commanders. The Combat Medic is a highly trained force multiplier. Medics have earned the respect of the Line throughout time. Today's Combat Medic is a noble professsion. They are ready to earn their place at home, in future conflicts, and disasters.

Past and present instructors of the Department of Combat Medic Training have authored this manual. We salute the Combat Medic and hope this will assist Combat Medics in understanding the profession.

"Soldier Medic / Warrior Spirit"

Patricia R. Hastings, COL, MC
SGM David J. Litteral, NREMT-P
Caron T. Wilbur, LTC, AN
Jeffrey S. Cain, MAJ, MC
Marshall Eidenberg, MAJ, MC
David S. Cahill, CSM (Ret.)

1 Triage

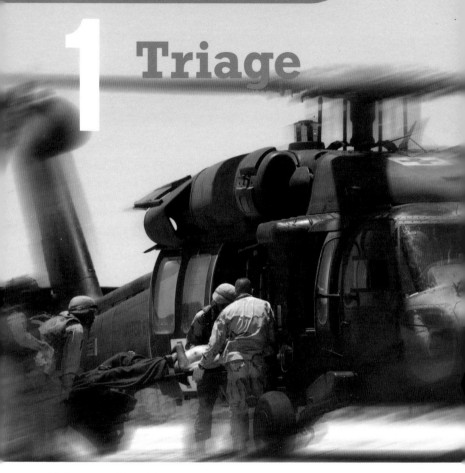

Triage Principles

- Do the greatest good for the greatest number of casualties.
- Employ the available resources in the most efficient way.
- Return key personnel to duty as quickly as possible.
- Continually reassess and re-triage.
- Move quickly.
- Do not second guess.
- The most experienced provider should triage.
- Plan, prepare, and train.

Triage Categories for Treatment

o Immediate: Implies the need for rapid intervention to save life, limb, or eyesight.

o Delayed: Implies significant injury or injuries that will require stabilization and treatment but are not expected to significantly deteriorate over several hours; this category of patients can safely wait until Immediate patients have been stabilized.

o Minimal: Implies the need for treatment, but the patient's condition is not expected to deteriorate over a day or so. These patients can help with self-aid or buddy-aid.

o Expectant: By definition, the patient is expected to die unless maximal resources are expended. It does *not* mean "no treatment." Rather, it means intensive, time-consuming treatment will be withheld until higher-priority patients are cared for. Comfort care should be given.

Triage Casualties

Performance Steps

1 Assess the situation.

o Sort the casualties and allocate treatment.
  ■ Assess and classify the casualties for the most efficient use of available medical personnel and supplies.
  ■ Give available treatment first to the casualties who have the best chance of survival.
  ■ A primary goal is to locate and return to duty troops with minor wounds. However, at no time should abandonment of a single casualty be considered.
  ■ Triage establishes the order of treatment, not whether treatment is given. It is usually the responsibility of the senior medical person.

o Determine the tactical situation and evaluate the environment.
  ■ Must casualties be transported to a more secure area for treatment?
  ■ What is the number and location of the injured and the severity of injuries?
  ■ What assistance (self-aid, buddy-aid, and medical personnel) is available?
  ■ What are the evacuation support capabilities and requirements?

> **note**
> Nuclear weapons exposure will not be used as criteria for sorting. Field experience with these injuries does not exist.

2 Assess the casualties and establish priorities for treatment.

o Immediate: Casualties whose conditions demand immediate treatment to save life, limb, or eyesight. This category has the highest priority.
- Airway obstruction
- Respiratory and cardiorespiratory distress from otherwise treatable injuries (for example, electrical shock, drowning, or chemical exposure)

A casualty with cardiorespiratory distress may not be classified "Immediate" on the battlefield. The casualty may be classified "Expectant," contingent upon such things as the situation, number of casualties, and support.

- Massive external bleeding
- Shock
- Burns on the face, neck, hands, feet, or perineum and genitalia

After all life- or limb-threatening conditions have been successfully treated, give no further treatment to the casualty until all other Immediate casualties have been treated. Salvage of life takes priority over salvage of limb.

o Chemical Immediate
- Presence of signs and symptoms of severe chemical agent poisoning
o Delayed: Casualties who have less risk of loss of life or limb if treatment is delayed.
- Open wounds of the chest without respiratory distress
- Open or penetrating abdominal injuries without shock
- Severe eye injuries without hope of saving eyesight
- Other open wounds
- Fractures
- Second and third degree burns (not involving the face, hands, feet, genitalia, and perineum) covering 20% or more of the total body surface area
- Presence of mild signs and symptoms of chemical agent poisoning
o Minimal: "Walking wounded," who can be treated by self-aid or buddy-aid.
- Minor lacerations and contusions
- Sprains and strains

- Minor combat stress problems
- First or second degree burns (not involving the face, hands, feet, genitalia, and perineum) covering under 20% of the total body surface area

○ Expectant: Casualties who are so critically injured that only complicated and prolonged treatment can improve life expectancy. This category is to be used only if resources are limited. If in doubt as to the severity of the injury, place the casualty in one of the other categories.
- Massive head injuries with signs of impending death
- Burns, mostly third degree, covering more than 85% of the total body surface area
- Presence of both chemical agent poisoning and life-threatening conventional injuries

note ————————————————————————

Provide ongoing supportive care if the time and condition permits; keep separate from other triage categorized casualties.

3 Record all treatment given on the Field Medical Card.

4 Establish MEDEVAC priorities by precedence category.

○ Urgent: Evacuation is required as soon as possible, but within 2 hours, to save life, limb, or eyesight. Generally, casualties whose conditions cannot be controlled and who have the greatest opportunity for survival are placed in this category.
- Cardiorespiratory distress
- Shock not responding to IV therapy
- Prolonged unconsciousness
- Head injuries with signs of increasing intracranial pressure
- Burns covering 20% to 85% of the total body surface area

○ Urgent Surgical: Evacuation is required for casualties who must receive far forward surgical intervention to save life and stabilize for further evacuation.
- Decreased circulation in the extremities
- Open chest and/or abdominal wounds with decreased blood pressure
- Penetrating wounds
- Uncontrollable bleeding or open fractures with severe bleeding
- Severe facial injuries

○ Priority: Evacuation is required within 4 hours or the casualty's condition could get worse and become an Urgent or Urgent Surgical condition. Generally, this category applies to any casualty whose condition is not stabilized or who is at risk of trauma-related complications.

- Closed-chest injuries, such as rib fractures without a flail segment, or other injuries that interfere with respiration
- Brief periods of unconsciousness
- Soft tissue injuries and open or closed fractures
- Abdominal injuries with no decreased blood pressure
- Eye injuries that do not threaten eyesight
- Spinal injuries
- Burns on the hands, face, feet, genitalia, or perineum even if under 20% of the total body surface area

○ Routine: Evacuation is required within 24 hours for further care. Immediate evacuation is not critical. Generally, this category covers casualties who can be controlled without jeopardizing their condition or who can be managed by the evacuating facility for up to 24 hours.

- Burns covering 20% to 80% of the total body surface area if the casualty is receiving and responding to IV therapy
- Simple fractures
- Open wounds, including chest injuries, without respiratory distress
- Psychiatric cases
- Terminal cases

○ Convenience: Evacuation by medical vehicle is a matter of convenience rather than necessity.

- Minor open wounds
- Sprains and strains
- Minor burns under 20% of total body surface area

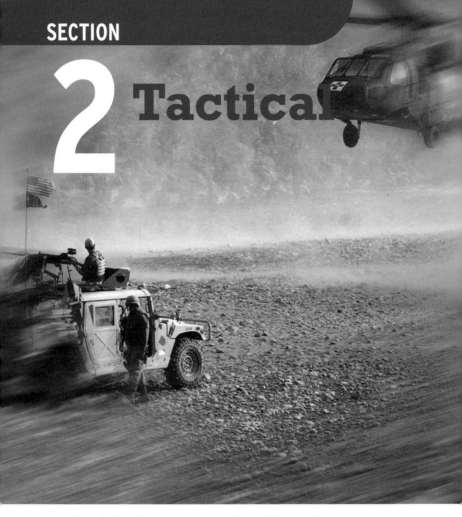

Tactical Medical Evaluation Checklist

Event	Responsibility	Go	No-Go
Planning/Predeployment Phase			
Combat Health Support Planning			
Medical threat assessment (*SRP status versus threat*)			
Determine medical assets (*organic, attached, air, ground, theater, JTF, host nation, ISB/FSB, etc.*)			
Gather higher HQ medical guidelines and requirements Familiarize with adjacent unit medical operations			
Submit medical RFIs Request maps, imagery, and medical intelligence			

Event	Responsibility	Go	No-Go
Understand the tactical commander's plan and concept of the operation			
Conduct a casualty estimation based off of the commander's concept of the operation by phase, objective, or event			
Determine key locations and designate a primary/alternate if appropriate: *unit objectives, Plt/Co/Bn CCPs, HLZs, AXPs, COB/EPW/NEO collection points, etc.*			
Determine the casualty flow from point of injury to tertiary fixed MTF (*key locations, distances, link-ups, etc.*)			
Plan for air CASEVAC (*dedicated assets, assets on-call, HLZs, request and launch methods, etc.*)			
Plan for ground CASEVAC (*dedicated assets, assets on-call, routes, AXPs, request and launch methods, etc.*)			
Determine medical communications requirements (*requesting and directing CASEVAC, casualty reporting, resupply requests, and medical call signs/frequencies on SOI*)			
Coordinate the casualty reporting/regulating system			
Synchronize medical events and systems into the unit's tactical synch matrix and execution checklist			
Determine Class VIII resupply requirements, methods, distribution, locations, packing lists, etc. (*synchronize with the unit's overall resupply system*)			
Determine preventive medicine requirements (*before, during and after the deployment*)			
Determine area medical support requirements at staging bases (*lab, x-ray, PM, etc.*)			
Schedule and coordinate CHS rehearsals with higher, adjacent, and subordinate elements (*CCP Ops, CASEVAC Ops, vehicle and aircraft loading/unloading*)			
Determine admin medical coverage requirements and integrate based on the tactical mission and SOPs			
Conduct Pre-Combat Checks			
Back-brief medical mission to higher medical authority, commanders, and leaders			
Draw/perform checks and maintenance on combat equipment *Weapons Protective masks* *Night vision Communications* *Mission specific*			

Event	Responsibility	Go	No-Go
Pack/re-pack trauma assault packs *Select appropriate aidbag or rucksack* *Ensure packing of recommended DOS stockage*			
Attend COMMEX *Ensure proper COMSEC* *Check/confirm frequencies and call signs*			
Verify and maintain copy of Battle Roster/Manifest *Co Sr Medics should have a Co Battle Roster* *Bn CCP should have a Bn or TF Battle Roster* *Infil/Exfil Manifests as appropriate*			
Check combat elements (Squads/Platoons/Companies) *All Soldiers - Individual Lifesaving Kits (ILSK)* *Combat Lifesavers - Combat Lifesavers Kit (CLSK),* *All Medics - Med supplies, drugs, and casualty cards*			
Verify dissemination of medical plan to the lowest level *CASEVAC procedures* *Medical locations*			
Rehearse and conduct CASEVAC drills with combat elements			
Pack/re-pack/stage medical resupply *Battalion Medical ISU-90/pallet* *Company deployment chests* *Reconfigure per mission specifics*			

Draw/perform checks on MEDSOV and quad
PMCS vehicle
Load required medical equipment:
  Litters (NATO, Sked, Isr)   Vehicle OVM/Tools
  O_2 Straps and tie-Downs
  Suction and BVM   Trauma Assault Packs
  Resupply bundles   Mission specifics
Gather operational required items
  Maps, imagery, overlays (routes, CCPs,
  HLZs, AXPs, AAs, fighting positions,
  objectives, phase lines)
  Communications SOI and COMSEC			

Conduct CHS Rehearsals			
CHS operations order/briefing (to all CHS participants) *Medical threat/intelligence* *Medical concept of the operation and casualty flow* *Key locations* *Requesting procedures (CASEVAC, resupply, etc.)* *Medical communications* *Casualty tracking*			

Event	Responsibility	Go	No-Go

CCP Operations
   CCP assembly, Security and movement plan
   Casualty movement and Aid and litter team plan
   Marking, Vehicle parking, Link-up procedures
   Casualty tracking and recording
   Triage, treatment, and management of casualties			

CASEVAC Drills
   Care under fire drills
   Air CASEVAC request and loading
   Ground CASEVAC request and loading			

Execution Phase			
Care Under Fire			
Return fire/control situation/recover casualty			
Provide immediate life-saving measures *Bleeding control*			
Communicate situation			
Tactical Field Care			
Evacuate casualty to CCP or secure location			
Conduct triage in a multiple casualty situation			
Conduct a rapid trauma assessment			
Treat life-threatening injuries/gain IV access			

Prep for evacuation
   Secure bandages, immobilize as required,
   prep evac-related equipment (litters, straps, etc.)			

Request evacuation and resupply (as required)			
Triage into a casualty collection point			
Perform detailed physical examination			
Definitive management of ABCs			
Request further evacuation and resupply			
Treat minor injuries (non-life-threatening) as time permits			
CCP Internal Evaluation/CASEVAC PREP			
CCP element assembly and link-up (75% assembled within 30 min of airdrop)			

CCP is established IAW the tactical timeline at
   the designated location. *If CCP is established*
   at alternate location or any other deviation in the
   plan, disseminate to units. Cover and concealment
   is utilized to the fullest extent possible.			

CCP security is established and maintained
   throughout op. *All pax maintain security/*
   situational awareness at all times.			

Event	Responsibility	Go	No-Go
CCP pax conduct appropriate noise, light, trash discipline at CCP sites for duration of op.			
Communications with C2 elements and units are established. *Execution checklist calls are made if required. Communication is established with company medics, 1SGs, and evac vehicles.*			
If marking devices are utilized, they are employed IAW SOP or the coordinated plan.			
Triage point is identified, marked, and used IAW SOP			
Casualties triaged into CCP by treatment category.			
Casualties recorded as they enter the CCP and reported to the TOC/CP/1SG/Head DACO as appropriate.			
Casualties are treated to the maximum available medical care standard as possible while in the CCP. *Casualties reassessed every 5 minutes or as the situation permits while in the CCP. Casualties are protected from the environment and covered/ concealed as much as the situation permits.*			
Evac from CCP is coordinated through appropriate C2 element			
EPW, COB, or NEO casualties are treated and evacuated IAW the Geneva Convention, SOP, or established plan			
Casualties have documentation/casualty card prior to evac from CCP (NLT evac from Bn level CCP)			
CCP personnel and casualties are extracted/recovered			
CASEVAC Operations			
Evac requests submitted IAW SOP or coordinated plan			
Vehicle movements coordinated through C2 elements			
CEPs, AXPs, HLZs, and link-ups are conducted IAW SOP or coordinated plan			
Air and ground evac ops are coordinated through C2 elements IAW SOP or coordinated plan			
Casualties evacuated by category (Urgent, Priority, Routine, or Convenience)			

Event	Responsibility	Go	No-Go
Casualty Treatment Evaluation (individual casualty trauma patient assessment)			
Determine responsiveness/level of consciousness			

Assess airway and breathing
   Assessment/patency
   Assures adequate ventilation, breathing rate and quality
   Manages injuries related to airway and breathing
   Manages airway (J-tube/nasopharyngeal/ suction/BVM/ET-tube/surgical airway)
   Administers oxygen if appropriate and available
   Manage C-spine* if indicated (as situation permits)			

Assess circulation
   Assess for and control life-threatening bleeding
   Assess pulse rate and quality
   Assess skin (color, temperature, and condition)			

Triages into evacuation or treatment category			
Conducts rapid or focused trauma assessment/ survey and treats life-threatening injuries appropriately			
Treat for shock			
Establishes vascular access (IV fluids or saline lock)			
Obtains baseline vital signs			

Obtains a patient history (Secondary survey as situation permits)
   SAMPLE history
   Self-aid/Buddy-aid/RFR care previously rendered?
   Previous interventions rendered?			

Conducts a detailed physical assessment
   (as situation permits)
   (inspect/palpate/auscultate OR pain/ blood/deformity)
   Assess head (scalp, ears, eyes/pupils, oro-nasal
   Assess neck (inspect, JVD, tracheal deviation)
   Assess chest (inspect, palpate, auscultate)
   Assess abdomen/pelvis/genitalia (palpate/auscultate)
   Assess extremities (pain, blood, deformity, pulses, motor/sensory)
   Assess posterior (sweep of back)			

Manages secondary injuries and wounds (as situation permits)			
Records patient information/treatment/interventions on casualty card (NLT Bn level CCP)			

Tactical Combat Casualty Care
Overview
As a soldier medic, you will be providing care in a variety of situations. The most stressful environment in which you will provide medical care is a combat situation. This lesson discusses the difference between garrison casualty care and combat casualty care.

- Medical training for combat medics is currently based on the principles for Emergency Medical Technicians (EMTs) and Basic and Advanced Trauma Life Support (BTLS and ATLS).
- These guidelines provide a standard systematic approach to the management of a trauma patient. This system works well in the setting of the civilian hospital emergency department. However, some of these principles may not be appropriate for the combat setting. In this block of instruction, we will discuss some significant differences in care provided in a combat setting.
  - The prehospital phase of care continues to be critically important. Most casualties in combat are the result of penetrating trauma, rather than the primarily blunt trauma seen in the civilian sector.
  - Up to 90% of combat deaths occur on the battlefield before a casualty reaches a medical treatment facility (MTF).
  - Factors influencing combat casualty care include the following:
    - Enemy fire (may prevent the treatment of casualties)
    - Medical equipment limitations (you only have what you carried in with you)
    - Widely variable evacuation time (from 30 minutes to several hours or days)
    - Tactical considerations (sometimes the mission will take precedence over medical care)
    - Casualty transportation (may or may not be available; air superiority must be achieved before any air evacuation assets will be deployed)

Stages of Care
In making the transition from civilian emergency care to the tactical setting, it is useful to consider the management of casualties that occur in a combat mission as being divided into three distinct phases:

- "Care Under Fire" is the care rendered by the medic at the scene of the injury while the medic and the casualty are still under effective hostile fire. Available medical equipment is limited to that carried by the individual soldier or the medic in his or her aid bag.

- "Tactical Field Care" is the care rendered by the medic once the medic and the casualty are no longer under effective hostile fire. It also applies to situations in which the injury has occurred on a mission, but there is no hostile fire. Available medical equipment is still limited to that being carried into the field by medical personnel. Time to evacuation to an MTF may vary considerably.
- "Combat Casualty Evacuation (CASEVAC) Care" is the care rendered once the casualty has been picked up by an aircraft, vehicle, or boat. Additional medical personnel and equipment may have been pre-staged and become available at this stage of casualty management.

Care Under Fire

- Medical personnel's firepower may be essential in obtaining tactical fire superiority. Attention to suppression of hostile fire may minimize the risk of injury to personnel and minimize additional injury to previously injured soldiers. (The best offense on the battlefield is tactical fire superiority.)
- Personnel may need to assist in returning fire instead of stopping to care for casualties. This includes the wounded who are still able to fight.
- Wounded soldiers who are unable to fight should lay flat and motionless if no cover is available or move as quickly as possible to any nearby cover.
- Medical personnel are limited; if they are injured, no other medical personnel will be available until the time of evacuation during the CASEVAC phase.
- No immediate management of the airway is necessary at this time because of the movement of the casualty to cover. Airway problems typically play a minimal role in combat casualties. Wound data from Korea and Vietnam indicate airway problems were only 1% to 6% of combat casualties, mostly from maxillofacial injuries.
- Control of hemorrhage, however, is important because injury to a major vessel can result in hypovolemic shock in a short time frame.

> **note**
>
> More than 2,500 deaths occurred in Vietnam secondary to hemorrhage from extremity wounds with no other injuries.

- Stop life-threatening external hemorrhage if tactically feasible:
  - Direct casualty to control hemorrhage by self aid if able.
  - Use a tourniquet for hemorrhage that is anatomically amenable to tourniquet application.
  - For hemorrhage that cannot be controlled with a tourniquet, apply HemCon dressing with pressure.

- Use of temporary tourniquets to stop the bleeding is essential in these types of casualties. If the casualty needs to be moved, as is usually the case, a tourniquet is the most reasonable initial choice to stop major bleeding. Ischemic damage to the limb is rare if the tourniquet is left in place for less than 1 hour, and tourniquets are often left in place for several hours during surgical procedures. In addition, the use of a temporary tourniquet may allow the injured soldier to continue to fight. Both the casualty and the medic are in grave danger while applying the tourniquet, and non-life-threatening bleeding should be ignored until the Tactical Field Care phase.
- Penetrating neck injuries do not require C-spine immobilization. Other neck injuries, such as falls from over 15 feet, fast roping injuries, or motor vehicle accidents (MVAs), may require C-spine immobilization unless the danger of hostile fire constitutes a greater threat in the judgment of the medic. Studies have shown that with penetrating neck injuries, only 1.4% of the injured would have benefited from C-spine immobilization. If C-collars are not available, a Sam splint can be used as a field-expedient C-collar.
- Litters may not be available for movement of casualties. Consider alternate methods to move casualties (e.g., ponchos, poleless litters, SKED litters, discarded doors, dragging, or manual carries). Smoke, combat support (CS), and vehicles may act as screens to assist in casualty movement.
- Do not attempt to salvage a casualty's rucksack unless it contains items critical to the mission.
- Take the patient's weapon and ammunition if possible to prevent the enemy from using it against you.
- Key points
  - Return fire as directed or required.
  - The casualty or casualties should also return fire if able.
  - Try to keep yourself from being shot.
  - Try to keep the casualty from sustaining any additional wounds.
  - Stop any life-threatening hemorrhage with a tourniquet.
  - Take the casualty with you when you leave.

Tactical Field Care

- The Tactical Field Care phase is distinguished from the Care Under Fire phase by a greater amount of time in which to provide care and a reduced level of hazard from hostile fire. The time available to render care may be quite variable. In some cases, tactical field care may consist of rapid treatment of wounds with the expectation of a re-engagement of hostile fire at any moment. In some circumstances there may be ample time to render whatever care is available in the field. The time to evacuation may be quite variable—from minutes to several hours.

- If a victim of a blast or penetrating injury is found without a pulse, respirations, or other signs of life, do not attempt CPR. Attempts to resuscitate trauma patients in arrest have been found to be futile even in the urban setting where the victim is in close proximity to a trauma center. On the battlefield, the cost of attempting CPR on casualties with what are inevitably fatal injuries is measured in additional lives lost because care is withheld from patients with less severe injuries and because medics are exposed to additional hazard from hostile fire during their attempts. Only in the case of non-traumatic disorders such as hypothermia, near drowning, or electrocution should CPR be considered.
- Patients with an altered level of consciousness should be disarmed immediately, both of weapons and grenades.
- Initial assessment consists of airway, breathing, and circulation.
  - Airway
    - Open the airway with a chin-lift or jaw-thrust maneuver in unconscious casualties and insert a nasopharyngeal airway (NPA) or Combitube. An NPA has the advantage of being better tolerated than an oropharyngeal airway (OPA) should the patient subsequently regain consciousness, and is less easily dislodged during patient transport. If the casualty needs a more advanced airway, the Combitube is the next recommended choice. Traditionally, the endotracheal tube (ETT) has been the gold standard for airway support. However, in combat the ETT has several disadvantages: (1) Many medics have never performed an intubation on a live patient or even a cadaver, (2) endotracheal intubation entails the use of white light on the battlefield, and (3) esophageal intubations are much less likely to be recognized on the battlefield and may result in fatalities. One study that examined first-time intubationists trained with manikins alone noted an initial success rate of only 42% in the ideal confines of the operating room with paralyzed patients. The Combitube is an effective airway designed for blind insertion. It is effective when placed in either the esophagus or the trachea. A study measuring effective placement of the Combitube noted it was successfully inserted 71% of the time for a first-line airway adjunct. The patient should also be placed in the recovery position.
    - If the casualty is unconscious and has an obstructed airway, and other airway techniques are not successful, perform a surgical cricothyroidotomy (with lidocaine if conscious). This may also be the airway of choice if maxillofacial injuries have disrupted the normal anatomy.
    - Oxygen is usually not available in this phase. Cylinders of compressed gas and the associated equipment for supplying the oxygen are too heavy to make their use in the field feasible.

- Breathing
  - Traumatic chest wall defects should be closed with an occlusive dressing without regard to venting one side of the dressing, because this is difficult to do in a combat setting. Alternatively, use an Asherman chest seal.
  - Progressive respiratory distress secondary to a unilateral chest trauma should be considered a tension pneumothorax and decompressed with a 14-gauge needle. The diagnosis in this setting should not rely on such typical signs as breath sounds, tracheal shift, and hyperresonance on percussion because these signs may not always be present, and even if they are, they may be exceedingly difficult to appreciate on the battlefield. Any patient with penetrating chest trauma will have some degree of hemopneumothorax as a result of the primary wound, and the additional trauma caused by a needle thoracostomy would not be expected to worsen the patient's condition. Chest tubes are not recommended in this phase of care because (1) they are not needed to provide initial treatment for a tension pneumothorax, (2) they are more difficult and time consuming for inexperienced personnel to use, especially in the absence of adequate light, (3) they are more likely to cause additional tissue damage and subsequent infection than a less traumatic procedure, and (4) no documentation has been found in the literature that demonstrated a benefit from tube thoracostomy performed by paramedical personnel on the battlefield. Chest tube placement does not cause re-inflation of the collapsed lung. In order for the lung to re-inflate, you must have suction to create a negative pressure in the chest cavity or positive pressure ventilation to blow the lung up from the inside.
- Bleeding
  - The medic should now address any significant bleeding sites not previously controlled. He or she should only remove the absolute minimum of the patient's clothing required to expose and treat injuries, both because of time constraints and the need to protect the patient from environmental extremes. Significant bleeding should be stopped as quickly as possible using a tourniquet as described previously. Once the tactical situation permits, consideration should be given to loosening the tourniquet and using direct pressure, a chitosan hemostatic dressing, or a hemostatic powder (e.g., QuikClot) to control any additional hemorrhage. Before releasing any tourniquet on a patient who has been resuscitated for hemorrhagic shock, ensure a positive response to resuscitation efforts (i.e., a peripheral pulse normal in character and normal mentation if there is no TBI).
- Intravenous access should be gained next. Although ATLS recommends starting two large-bore (14- or 16-gauge) IVs, a single 18-gauge

catheter is preferred in the field setting because of the ease of starting and the conservation of supplies. Heparin or saline lock-type access tubing should be used unless the patient needs immediate fluid resuscitation. Flushing the saline lock every 2 hours will usually suffice to keep it open without the need to use heparinized solution. Medics should ensure that the IV is not started distal to a significant wound. If unable to start a peripheral IV, consider starting a sternal intraosseous (IO) line to provide fluids. The F.A.S.T.1 device is available, which allows the puncture of the manubrium of the sternum and administration of fluids at rates similar to IVs. Stethoscopes and blood pressure cuffs are rarely available or useful to the front-line medic in the typically noisy and chaotic battlefield environment. A palpable radial pulse and normal mentation are adequate and tactically relevant resuscitation endpoints to either start or stop fluid resuscitation. Both can be adequately assessed in noisy and chaotic situations without mechanical devices.

- Fluids
  - 1,000 mL (2.4 lb) of Ringer's lactate will expand the intravascular volume 250 mL within 1 hour.
  - 500 mL of 6% hetastarch (trade name Hextend, weighs 1.3 lb) will expand the intravascular volume by 800 mL within 1 hour. One 500-mL bag of Hextend is functionally equivalent to three 1,000-mL bags of lactated Ringer's, although there is more than a 51 to 2 advantage in the overall weight-to-benefit ratio (1.3 lb to 7.2 lb, respectively). This expansion is sustained for at least 8 hours.
  - The first consideration in selecting a resuscitation fluid is whether to use a crystalloid or colloid. Crystalloids are fluids such as Ringer's lactate or normal saline in which sodium is the primary osmotically active solute. Because sodium eventually distributes throughout the entire extracellular space, most of the fluids in crystalloid solutions remain in the intravascular space for only a limited time. Colloids are solutions in which the primary osmotically active molecules are of greater molecular weight and do not readily pass through the capillary walls into the interstitium. These solutions are retained in the intravascular space for much longer periods of time than crystalloids. In addition, the oncotic pressure of colloid solutions may result in an expansion of the blood volume that is greater than the amount infused.
  - Algorithm for fluid resuscitation
    - Superficial wounds (which account for more than 50% of the injured): No immediate IV fluids are needed; oral fluids should be encouraged.

- Any significant extremity or truncal wound (neck, chest, abdomen, and pelvis) with or without obvious blood loss or hypotension: If the soldier is coherent and has a palpable radial pulse, blood loss has likely stopped. Start a saline lock, hold fluids, and re-evaluate as frequently as the situation allows.
- Significant blood loss from any wound, and the soldier has no radial pulse or is not coherent: *Stop the bleeding* by whatever means available—tourniquet, direct pressure, hemostatic dressing (HemCon), hemostatic powder (QuikClot). However, greater than 90% of hypotensive casualties suffer from truncal injuries, which are unmanageable by these resuscitative measures. (Patients will have lost a minimum of 1,500 mL of blood or 30% of their circulating volume.) After hemorrhage is controlled to the extent possible, start 500 mL of Hextend. If mental status improves and radial pulse returns, maintain saline lock and hold fluids. If no response is seen within 30 minutes, give an additional 500 mL of Hextend and monitor vital signs. If no response is seen after 1,000 mL of Hextend, consider triaging supplies and attention to more salvageable casualties. Remember, this amount is equivalent to more than 6 liters of Ringer's lactate. Because of coagulation concerns, no casualty should receive more than 1,000 mL of Hextend.
- Uncontrolled hemorrhage (thoracic or intra-abdominal): Rapid evacuation and surgical intervention are needed. If this is not possible, then determine the number of casualties versus the amount of available fluid. If supplies are limited or casualties are numerous, determine if fluid resuscitation is recommended. A number of studies involving uncontrolled hemorrhage models have clearly established that aggressive fluid resuscitation in the setting of unrepaired vascular injury is either of no benefit or results in an increase in blood loss or mortality when compared with no fluid resuscitation or hypotensive resuscitation. Several studies noted that only after uncontrolled hemorrhage was stopped did fluid resuscitation prove to be of benefit. Continued efforts to resuscitate must be weighed against logistical and tactical considerations and the risk of incurring further casualties. If a casualty with TBI is unconscious and has no peripheral pulse, resuscitate to restore the radial pulse.

○ Dress wounds to prevent further contamination and help hemostasis. Check for additional wounds (exit wounds) because the high-velocity projectiles from modern assault rifles may tumble and take erratic courses when traveling through tissues, often leading to exit sites remote from the entry wound. Only remove enough clothing to expose wounds.

○ Prevention of Hypothermia
  ■ Minimize casualty's exposure to the elements. Keep protective gear on or with the casualty, if feasible.
  ■ Replace wet clothing with dry, if possible.

- Apply Ready-Heat blanket to torso.
- Wrap in Blizzard Rescue blanket.
- Put Thermo-Lite Hypothermia Prevention System cap on the casualty's head, under his/her helmet.
- Apply additional interventions as needed/available.
- If mentioned gear is not available, use dry blankets, poncho liners, sleeping bags, body bags, or anything that will retain heat and keep the casualty dry.

○ Monitoring
- Pulse oximetry should be available as an adjunct to clinical monitoring. Readings may be misleading in the settings of shock or marked hypothermia.

○ Pain control
- If the patient is able to fight: These medications should be carried by the combatant and self-administered as soon as possible after the wound is sustained:
  - Mobic 15 mg PO qd
  - Tylenol 650 mg bi-layer caplet, 2 PO q8h
- Unable to fight:

> **note**
>
> Have naloxone readily available whenever administering opiates.

  - Does not otherwise require IV/IO access:
    - Oral transmucosal fentanyl citrate 400 μg transbuccally.
      - Recommend taping lozenge on a stick to casualty's finger as an added safety measure.
      - Reassess in 15 minutes.
      - Add second lozenge, in other cheek, as necessary to control severe pain.
      - Monitor for respiratory depression.
  - IV/IO obtained:
    - Morphine sulfate 5 mg IV/IO
      - Reassess in 10 minutes.
      - Repeat dose q 10 min as necessary to control severe pain.
      - Monitor for respiratory depression.
    - Promethazine 25 mg IV/IO/IM q 4h, for synergistic analgesic effect, and as a counter to potential nausea.
  - Soldiers should avoid aspirin and other nonsteroidal anti-inflammatory medicines while in a combat zone because of their detrimental effects on hemostasis.

○ Fractures should be splinted as circumstances allow, insuring pulse checks before and after splinting.

○ Antibiotics: recommended for all open combat wounds.
  ■ If able to take PO:
    • Gatifloxacin 400 mg PO qd
  ■ If unable to take PO (shock, unconsciousness):
    • Cefotetan 2 g IV (slow push over 3–5 minutes) or IM q12h *or*
    • Ertapenem 1 g IV or IM q24h
  ■ In soldiers who are awake and alert, gatifloxacin 400 mg orally every day is an acceptable regimen. Each individual soldier is issued this medication prior to deployment. In unconscious patients, use cefotetan 2 g IV push over 3 to 5 minutes, which may be repeated at 12-hour intervals until evacuation.
  ■ In personnel with allergies to fluoroquinolones or cephalosporins, consider other broad-spectrum antibiotics in the planning phase.
  ■ Communicate with the patient, if possible:
    • Encourage, reassure.
    • Explain care.
  ■ Document clinical assessments, treatments rendered, and changes in casualty's status. Forward this information with the casualty to the next level of care.
○ Key points
  ■ Airway management
    • Perform a chin-lift or jaw-thrust maneuver.
    • Unconscious patient without an airway obstruction: Insert NPA or Combitube; place patient in the recovery position.
    • Unconscious patient with an airway obstruction: Perform cricothyroidotomy.
    • Cervical spine immobilization is not necessary for penetrating neck or head trauma.
  ■ Breathing: If a casualty has a unilateral penetrating chest wound and progressive respiratory distress, assume a tension pneumo-thorax and decompress the chest with needle decompression.
  ■ Bleeding: Control any bleeding with a tourniquet, direct pressure, hemostatic dressing, or hemostatic powder (e.g., QuikClot).
  ■ IV: Start an 18-gauge IV or saline lock. Consider sternal IO infusion if unable to start IV.
  ■ Fluid resuscitation
    • Controlled hemorrhage without shock: No fluids necessary.
    • Controlled hemorrhage with shock: Hextend, up to 1,000 mL.
    • Uncontrolled (intra-abdominal or thoracic) hemorrhage: Rapid evacuation if possible. Remember, do not administer more than 1,000 mL of Hextend to any one casualty.
  ■ Inspect and dress wounds; check for additional wounds.
  ■ Pain management as necessary. If able to fight: Toradol 10 mL PO with acetaminophen 1,000 mg PO Q 6 hours. If unable to fight:

Morphine 5 mg IV, wait 10 minutes; repeat as necessary. Medics trained in the use of morphine must also be trained in the use of naloxone.

- Splint fractures and recheck pulses after splinting.
- Antibiotics: Gatifloxacin 400 mg orally every day if patient is awake and alert. If patient is unconscious, cefotetan 2 g slow IV push (over 3 to 5 minutes) may be repeated every 12 hours until evacuation.
- Resuscitation on the battlefield for victims of blast or penetrating trauma who have no pulse, no respirations, and no signs of life will not be successful and should not be attempted.
- Soldiers with an altered level of consciousness should be disarmed immediately.

Combat Casualty Evacuation Care

○ The term "CASEVAC care" differs significantly from the traditional term "medical evacuation (MEDEVAC)." The Army and the Navy use the term "MEDEVAC" when describing the evacuation of wounded combat personnel from the field with medical assets. The Air Force considers the term "MEDEVAC" to apply to the medical evacuation of a stable patient from one medical facility to another. The term "CASEVAC" is the recommended term when discussing the initial management of combat casualty evacuation from the battlefield with no medical assets.

○ There are only minor differences in the care provided in the CASEVAC phase versus the Tactical Field Care phase.
- Additional medical personnel may accompany the evacuation asset and assist the medic on the ground. This may be important for the following reasons:
  - The medic may be among the casualties.
  - The medic may be dehydrated, hypothermic, or otherwise debilitated.
  - The EVAC asset's medical equipment may need to be prepared prior to evacuation.
  - There may be multiple casualties that exceed the medic's capability to care for simultaneously.
- Additional medical equipment can be brought with the evacuation asset to augment the equipment the medic currently has. This equipment may include laryngeal mask airway (LMA), endotracheal intubation equipment, or electronic monitoring equipment capable of measuring a patient's blood pressure, pulse, and pulse oximetry.
  - Oxygen should be available during this phase.
  - Ringer's lactate at a rate of 250 mL per hour for patients not in shock should help to reverse dehydration, and blood products may be available during this phase.
  - Spinal immobilization is not necessary for casualties with penetrating trauma.

- Prevention of hypothermia
  - Minimize casualty's exposure to the elements. Keep protective gear on or with the casualty, if feasible.
  - Continue Ready-Heat blanket, Blizzard Rescue blanket, and Thermo-Lite cap.
  - Utilize the Thermal Angel or other possible fluid warmers on all IV sites, if possible.
  - Protect the casualty from wind if doors must be kept open.
- Pneumatic antishock garment (PASG) may be useful for stabilizing pelvic fractures and controlling pelvic and abdominal bleeding. Its application and extended use must be carefully monitored. It is contraindicated for casualties with thoracic and brain injuries.
- Document clinical assessment, treatments rendered, and changes in casualty's status. Forward this information with the casualty to the next level of care.

○ Key points
- Airway: Same as Tactical Field Care.
- Breathing: Same as Tactical Field Care, except add oxygen.
- Bleeding: Consider removing tourniquets and using direct pressure, hemostatic dressings, or hemostatic powder (e.g., QuikClot) to control bleeding.
- IV: Start 18-gauge IV or saline lock, if not already done. Consider sternal IO access if unable to start IV.
- Fluid resuscitation: Same as Tactical Field Care, except add Ringer's lactate at 250 mL per hour to reverse dehydration, if necessary. Blood products may be available in this phase.
- Monitoring: Institute electronic monitoring of heart rate, blood pressure, and oxygen saturation.
- Inspect and dress wounds (same as Tactical Field Care).
- Check for additional wounds (same as Tactical Field Care).
- Analgesia: Same as Tactical Field Care.
- Splint fractures (same as Tactical Field Care).
- Antibiotics: Same as Tactical Field Care.

Summary

Medical care during combat operations differs significantly from the care provided in the civilian community. New concepts in hemorrhage control, fluid resuscitation, analgesia, and antibiotics are important means of providing the best possible care for our combat soldiers. These timely interventions will be the mainstay in decreasing the number of combat fatalities on the battlefield.

Anaphylactic Shock

Performance Steps

Anaphylactic reactions occur within minutes or even seconds after contact with the substance to which the casualty is allergic. Reactions occur in the skin, respiratory system, and circulatory system.

1 Check the casualty for signs and symptoms of anaphylactic shock.

- Skin
  - Flushed or ashen
  - Burning or itching
  - Edema (swelling), especially in the face, tongue, or airway
  - Urticaria (hives) spreading over the body
  - Marked swelling of the lips and eyes
- Respiratory system
  - Tightness or pain in the chest
  - Sneezing and coughing
  - Wheezing, stridor, or difficulty in breathing (dyspnea)
  - Respiratory failure
- Circulatory system
  - Weak, rapid pulse
  - Hypotension
  - Dizziness or fainting
  - Coma

2 Transport the casualty to the aid station.

▼ WARNING

Do not attempt to transport the casualty to an aid station unless the station can be reached within 4 minutes. Otherwise, start supportive treatment immediately and transport the casualty as soon as possible.

3 Open the airway, if necessary.

note

In cases of airway obstruction from severe glottic edema, a cricothyroidotomy may be necessary.

4 Administer high-concentration oxygen.

5 Administer epinephrine.

o Administer 0.5 mL of epinephrine, 1:1000 solution, subcutaneously (SQ) or intramuscularly (IM).

> **note**
>
> Annotate the time of injection on the Field Medical Card (FMC).

o Additional epinephrine may be required as anaphylaxis progresses. Additional incremental doses may be administered every 5 to 15 minutes in accordance with local standard operating procedures.

6 Initiate an IV.

> **note**
>
> If the anaphylaxis is due to an insect bite or sting on an extremity, remove the stinger as quickly as possible. This is best accomplished by scraping with a credit card or blade. A constricting band should be applied 2 to 3 inches above and below the site. The band should be loose enough to allow arterial flow but tight enough to restrict venous circulation. A distal pulse must be palpable. Keep the limb immobilized and the patient still.

7 Provide supportive measures for the treatment of shock, respiratory failure, circulatory collapse, or cardiac arrest.

o Infuse additional IV fluid if blood pressure continues to drop.
o Position the patient in the supine position with legs elevated if injuries permit.
o Perform rescue breathing, if necessary.
o Administer external chest compressions, if necessary.

8 Check the casualty's vital signs every 3 to 5 minutes until the casualty is stable.

9 Record the procedure on the appropriate form.

10 Evacuate the casualty, providing supportive measures en route.

Burn Injury

Performance Steps

1 Determine the cause of the burns.

o Assess the scene.
o Question the casualty and/or bystanders.
o Determine if the casualty has been exposed to smoke, steam, or combustible products.
o Determine if the cause was open flame, hot liquid, chemicals, or electricity.
o Determine whether the casualty was struck by lightning.

> **note**
>
> If the burn was caused by an explosion or lightning, the casualty may also have been thrown some distance from the original spot of the incident. He or she may therefore have associated internal injuries, fractures, or spinal injuries.

2 Stop the burning process.

o Thermal burns
  - Have the casualty *stop*, *drop*, and *roll*.
    - Do not permit the casualty to run, because this will fan the flames.
    - Do not permit the casualty to stand, because the flames may be inhaled or the hair ignited.
    - Place the casualty on the ground or floor and smother the casualty in a blanket.
  - Remove all smoldering clothing and articles that retain heat, if possible.
  - Cut away clothing to expose the burned area.

> **CAUTION**
>
> Do not remove clothing that is stuck to the burned area. If the clothing and skin are still hot, cover with a burn dressing, if available.

o Electrical burns
  - Turn off the current, if possible (contact appropriate personnel to shut off electricity).

▼ WARNING

Do not directly touch a casualty receiving a shock. To do so will conduct the current to you.

▼ WARNING

Electrical shock may cause the casualty to go into cardiac arrhythmia or arrest. Initiate CPR as appropriate. Casualties of lightning strikes may require prolonged CPR and extended respiratory support.

○ Chemical burns

▼ WARNING

A chemical will burn as long as it is in contact with the skin.

■ Flush the area of contact immediately with water. Do not delay flushing by removing the casualty's clothing first.

> **note**
>
> If a solid chemical, such as lime, has been spilled on the casualty, brush it off before flushing. A dry chemical is activated by contact with water and will cause more damage to the skin.

■ Flush with cool water for a minimum of 20 minutes while removing contaminated clothing or other articles.

> **note**
>
> (1) Flush longer for alkali burns because they penetrate deeper and cause more severe injury. (2) Many chemicals have a delayed reaction. They will continue to cause injury even though the casualty no longer feels pain.

▼ WARNING

Do not use a hard blast of water. Extreme water pressure can add mechanical injury to the skin.

○ White phosphorus burns

note

White phosphorus (WP) will stick to the skin and continue to burn until it is deprived of air. WP burns are usually multiple and deep, usually producing second and third degree burns.

- Deprive the WP of oxygen.
  - Submerge the entire area.
  - Cover the affected area with a moistened cloth, if available, or mud.
- Remove superficial WP particles from the skin by brushing with a wet cloth or using a forceps, stick, or knife.

3 Open and maintain an airway, if necessary.

note

For inhalation injuries, as long as 30 to 40 minutes may elapse before edema obstructs the airway and respiratory distress is noted.

○ Check for signs and symptoms of inhalation injury.
  - Facial burns
  - Singed eyebrows, eyelashes, and/or nasal hairs
  - Carbon deposits and/or redness in the mouth and/or oropharynx
  - Sooty carbon deposits in the sputum
  - Hoarseness, noisy inhalation, brassy-sounding cough, or dyspnea
○ Check for signs and symptoms of carbon monoxide poisoning in enclosed-space fires.
  - Dizziness, nausea, and/or headache
  - Cyanosis
  - Tachycardia or tachypnea
  - Respiratory distress or arrest
○ Administer humidified oxygen at a high flow rate.

4 Determine the percentage of body surface area (BSA) burned.

○ Cut the casualty's clothing away from the burned areas.
○ Determine the percentage of BSA burned using the Rule of Nines (**Figure 1**).

5 Determine the degree of the burns.

○ First degree
  - Superficial skin only
  - Red and painful, like a sunburn

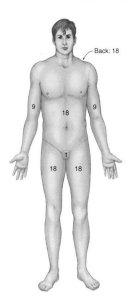

Figure 1 Rule of Nines, showing distribution of body surface area by anatomic parts in the adult.

- o Second degree
  - ▪ Partial thickness of the skin
  - ▪ Penetrates the skin deeper than first degree
  - ▪ Blisters and pain
  - ▪ Some subcutaneous edema
- o Third degree
  - ▪ Damage to or the destruction of a full thickness of skin
  - ▪ Involves underlying muscles, bones, or other structures
  - ▪ Skin may look leathery, dry, and discolored (charred, brown, or white)
  - ▪ Nerve ending destruction causes a lack of pain
  - ▪ Massive fluid loss
  - ▪ Clotted blood vessels may be visible under the burned skin
  - ▪ Subcutaneous fat may be visible

CAUTION

(1) Check for entry and exit burns when treating electrical burns and lightning strikes. (2) The amount of injured tissue in an electrical burn is usually far more extensive than the appearance of the wound would indicate. Although the burn wounds may be small, severe damage may occur to deeper tissues. (High voltage can destroy skin and muscles to such an extent that amputation may eventually be necessary.)

Table 1 Parkland Formula for Estimating Adult Burn Patient Resuscitation Fluid Needs

4 mL (cc) × Weight (kg) × % BSA = cc of Ringer's lactate for first 24 hours
Give half in the first 8 hours postburn, the rest over the next 16 hours.

6 Treat those casualties who have second- or third-degree burns of 20% BSA or more for shock.

○ Initiate treatment for hypovolemic shock.
○ Keep the casualty flat.
○ Initiate an IV.
  ■ Use Ringer's lactate, if available. Normal saline is the second fluid of choice.
  ■ Use a large-gauge (no. 16 or 18) needle.
  ■ Initiate the IV in an unburned area, if possible.
  ■ Use a large peripheral vein.

> **note**
>
> The presence of overlying burned skin should not deter the use of an accessible vein. The upper extremities are preferable to lower extremities.

○ Infuse fluids for a casualty based on fluid replacement calculations (see the following method and **Table 1**).
  ■ Calculate the casualty's body weight in kilograms (kg).
    • Determine or estimate the casualty's body weight in pounds.
    • Divide the casualty's body weight by 2.2. For example, if the casualty weighs about 165 pounds, the calculation is 165/2.2 = 75 kg.
  ■ Calculate the amount of fluid to infuse per hour for the next 8 hours.
    • Determine the percentage of BSA burned using the Rule of Nines. For example, assume that the casualty's BSA burned is 36%.
    • Multiply 1 mL of fluid (1.00 cc) by the percentage of BSA burned. For our example, this is 1.00 cc × 36 = 36 cc.
    • Multiply the resulting figure by the casualty's weight, in kilograms. For our example: 36 cc × 75 kg = 2,700 cc. The casualty will require this much fluid over the next 8 hours.
    • Divide the figure obtained in the previous calculation by 8 to determine the amount of fluid to give per hour. For our example, the calculation is 2700/8 = 337.5, rounded to 338 cc of fluid per hour (cc/hr).

■ Assess the circulatory blood volume.

> **note**
>
> Urine output is a reliable guide to assess circulating blood volume.

■ Measure the casualty's urine output in cc per hour.
■ Adjust the IV fluid flow to maintain 30 to 50 cc of urine output per hour.

7 Stabilize the casualty and perform a secondary assessment.

o Measure and record the casualty's vital signs.
o Assess the casualty for associated injuries.
o Check the distal circulation by checking pulses in all extremities.

8 Remove potentially constricting items such as rings and bracelets.

> **CAUTION**
>
> The swelling of burns on extremities can cause a tourniquet-like effect, and the swelling of a burned throat can impair breathing.

9 Dress the burns.

o Apply a dry sterile dressing to the burns.

> **CAUTION**
>
> Do not put ointment on the burns, and do not break blisters.

o Cover extensive burns with a sterile sheet, if available, or clean linen.

10 Administer oxygen, if available.

11 Record the treatment given.

12 Evacuate the casualty.

Cold Injury

Performance Steps

1 Recognize the signs and symptoms of cold injuries.

o Chilblain is caused by repeated prolonged exposure of bare skin to low temperatures from 60°F (15.6°C) down to 32°F (0°C).
■ Acutely red, swollen, hot, tender, and/or itching skin
■ Surface lesions with shedding of dead tissue, or bleeding lesions

- Frostbite is caused by exposure of the skin to cold temperatures that are usually below 32°F (0°C) depending on the windchill factor, length of exposure, and adequacy of protection.

  note

  The onset of frostbite is signaled by a sudden blanching of the skin of the nose, ears, cheeks, fingers, or toes followed by a momentary tingling sensation.

- Superficial (first and second degree)
  - Redness of the skin in light-skinned individuals, and grayish coloring of the skin in dark-skinned individuals; decreased sensation initially, followed by intense burning, followed by a flaky sloughing of the skin in several days.
  - Blister formation 24 to 36 hours after exposure followed by sheet-like sloughing of the superficial skin (second degree). Blister formation may be clear or discolored.
- Deep
  - Loss of feeling
  - Pale, yellow, waxy look if the affected area is unthawed
  - Solid feel of the frozen tissue
  - Blister formation 12 to 36 hours after exposure unless rewarming is rapid
  - Appearance of red-violet discoloration 1 to 5 days after the injury

    note

    Gangrene and residual nerve damage will result without proper treatment.

- Generalized hypothermia is caused by prolonged exposure to low temperatures, especially with wind and wet conditions, and it may be caused by immersion in cold water.

  CAUTION

  With generalized hypothermia, the entire body has cooled, with the core temperature below 95°F (35°C). This is a medical emergency.

- Moderate hypothermia

  note

  Moderate hypothermia should be suspected in any chronically ill person who is found in an environment of less than 50°F (10°C).

- Conscious, but usually apathetic or lethargic
- Shivering, with pale, cold skin; slurred speech; poor muscle coordination; faint pulse
  - Severe hypothermia
    - Unconscious or stuporous
    - Ice-cold skin
    - Inaudible heart beat or irregular heart rhythm
    - Unobtainable blood pressure
    - Unreactive pupils
    - Very slow respirations
- Immersion syndrome (immersion foot, trench foot, and trench hand) is caused by fairly long (hours to days) exposure of the feet or hands to wet conditions at temperatures from about 50°F (10°C) down to 32°F (0°C).
  - First phase (anesthetic)
    - There is decreased sensation, and the affected area feels cold.
    - The pulse is weak at the affected area.
  - Second phase (reactive hyperemic)
    - Limbs feel hot and/or burning and have shooting pains.
  - Third phase (vasospastic)
    - Affected area is pale.
    - Cyanosis is evident.
    - Pulse strength decreases.
  - Check for blisters, swelling, redness, heat, hemorrhage, or gangrene.
- Snow blindness
  - Scratchy feeling in the eyes as if from sand or dirt
  - Watery eyes
  - Pain, possibly as late as 3 to 5 hours after exposure
  - Reluctance or inability to open eyes

2 Treat the cold injury.

- Chilblain
  - Apply local rewarming within minutes.
  - Protect lesions (if present) with dry sterile dressings.

    CAUTION

    Do not treat chilblains with ointments.

- Frostbite
  - Apply local rewarming using body heat.

    CAUTION

    Avoid thawing the affected area if it is possible that the injury may refreeze before reaching the treatment center.

- Loosen or remove constricting clothing and remove jewelry.
- Increase insulation and exercise the entire body as well as the affected body part or parts.

CAUTION

Do not massage the skin or rub anything on the frozen parts.

- Move the casualty to a sheltered area, if possible.
- Protect the affected area from further cold or trauma.
- Evacuate the casualty.

note

For frostbite of a lower extremity, evacuate the casualty by litter, if possible.

CAUTION

Do not allow the casualty to use tobacco or alcohol.

○ Generalized hypothermia
- Moderate hypothermia
  - Remove the casualty from the cold environment.
  - Replace wet clothing with dry clothing.
  - Cover the casualty with insulating material or blankets.
  - If available, apply heating pads to the casualty's armpits, groin, and abdomen.

note

If far from a medical treatment facility and if the situation and facilities permit, immerse the casualty in a tub of 104°F (40°C) water; keep extremities out of the water, allowing the central core to warm first. This is a last-ditch method for warming; every attempt should be made to evacuate the casualty.

  - If available, slowly give sugar and sweet, warm fluids.

CAUTION

Do not give the casualty alcohol.

  - Wrap the casualty from head to toe.
  - Evacuate the casualty lying down.

■ Severe hypothermia

CAUTION

Handle the casualty very gently.

· Cut away wet clothing and replace it with dry clothing.
· Maintain the airway.
  ■ Administer oxygen if trained personnel and equipment are available.
  ■ Assist with ventilation if the casualty's respiration rate is less than 5 breaths per minute.

note

Do not use artificial airways or suctioning devices.

CAUTION

Do not hyperventilate the casualty. Keep the rate of artificial ventilation at approximately 8 to 10 breaths per minute.

· Monitor the patient's pulse. If none is detected, apply automated external defibrillator, if available. Begin CPR. IV fluids should be warmed to 104°F (40°C) before administration.
· Handle the casualty gently; rough handling can precipitate cardiac arrhythmias.

note

The treatment of moderate hypothermia is aimed at preventing further heat loss and rewarming the casualty as rapidly as possible. Rewarming a casualty with severe hypothermia is critical to saving his or her life, but the kind of care that rewarming requires is nearly impossible to carry out in the field. Evacuate the casualty promptly to a medical treatment facility. Use stabilizing measures en route.

■ Immersion syndrome
  · Dry the affected part immediately and gradually rewarm it in warm air.

Never massage the skin. After rewarming the affected part, it may become swollen, red, and hot. Blisters usually form due to tissue damage.

- Protect the affected part from trauma and secondary infection.
- Elevate the affected part.
- Evacuate the casualty as soon as possible.
- Snow blindness: Cover the eyes with a dark cloth and evacuate the casualty to a medical treatment facility.

Dental Emergencies

Avulsed Tooth

- Introduction: Tooth completely removed from socket.
- Subjective (symptoms): History of trauma or severe dental caries; may present with tooth in hand.
- Objective (signs): Visible space or empty socket.
- Assessment: Look for other injury if related to trauma.
- Plan
  - If tooth has been saved, transport avulsed tooth in any clean liquid medium (saline, milk, or saliva). Do not let tooth dry out. Gently rinse tooth with 0.9% normal saline. Do not scrape off any debris or attempt to scale the tooth.
  - Administer local anesthetic, if available, and you are trained to do so.
  - Replace tooth into its socket.
  - If blood clot prevents tooth placement, rinse socket with saline to remove blood clot.
  - Splint the tooth to adjacent teeth with dental wires, heavy monofilament, intermediate restorative material (IRM)/ cotton fiber splint, or a glass ionomer splint.
  - Provide pain relief. Use acetaminophen or ibuprofen for mild pain. Use acetaminophen with codeine for more severe pain.

CAUTION

Do not use aspirin products if excessive bleeding is noted.

  - Administer antibiotic regimen.
  - Evacuate for consultant care.

> **note**
> ─────────────────────────────────────
>
> A partially avulsed tooth that is repositioned is usually
> permanently retained. A completely avulsed tooth may
> be permanently retained if replaced in the socket with
> minimal handling in less than one hour. When the
> replacement time exceeds one hour, the long-term
> retention rate drops and root resorption usually occurs.

Dental Caries ("Cavities")

- Subjective (symptoms): Intermittent or continuous pain, usually intense.
  Heat, cold, sweet, acid, or salty substances may worsen the pain.
- Objective (signs): Finding the offending tooth may be difficult, but it
  will usually be grossly decayed, with the carious enamel and dentin
  area discolored. The tooth will be tender and sensitive to heat and
  cold. Tapping the tooth with an instrument will usually elicit pain.
  When conducting a thermal test, use a normal tooth as a basis for
  comparison. Check vitality: Pain upon touching dentin indicates
  vitality. A vital tooth will give a painful response to cold.
- Assessment (differential diagnosis): Caries in vital tooth versus dead
  tooth.
- Plan
  - Primary: Remove caries and place a temporary restoration. Local
    anesthetic may be necessary before applying a temporary restoration.
  - Alternate: For teeth that are still vital, eugenol (IRM liquid) is an
    agent that will temporarily soothe hyperemic pulp tissue if used
    indirectly (i.e., not in direct contact with the pulp). If a mixture of
    zinc oxide and eugenol is applied directly to vital pulp, it will kill the
    pulp. A dental officer must give definitive care in the near future.
  - Patient education: Do not chew on the treated tooth.

Luxated (Dislocated) Tooth

- Introduction: A tooth moved from normal position.
- Subjective (symptoms): History of trauma or biting into hard object.
- Objective (signs): Visibly malpositioned tooth.
- Assessment: Look for other injury if related to trauma.
- Plan: Administer local anesthetic if available and you are trained to
  do so. Manually reposition tooth into normal occlusal scheme. Stabi-
  lize tooth with gentle pressure during splinting procedure. Splint to
  adjacent teeth with wire, heavy monofilament fishing line, an
  IRM/cotton fiber splint, or glass ionomer splint.

Tooth/Crown Fractures

- Introduction: Anterior (front) teeth are particularly susceptible to injuries that result in fracture of the crown.
- Subjective (symptoms): History of trauma or biting hard object; feels jagged tooth edge; finds tooth fragment; sensitivity to heat and/or cold.
- Objective (signs): Visibly broken or cracked tooth.
- Assessment: Look for other injury if related to trauma.
- Plan
  - Simple fractures of the crown involving little or no dentin: Smooth the rough edges of the tooth with an emery board or small flat file.
  - Extensive fractures of the crown involving considerable dentin but not the pulp
    - Wash the tooth with warm saline.
    - Isolate and dry the tooth with cotton gauze or rolls.
    - Then cover the exposed dentin using one of several methods:
      - Cover the exposed dentin with (IRM) zinc oxide-eugenol paste (it is difficult to achieve retention on anterior fractures). An aluminum crown, trimmed and contoured to avoid lacerating the gingiva, can be filled with this paste and placed over the tooth.
      - Incorporate cotton fibers into a mix of zinc oxide and eugenol (the fibers give additional strength) and place this over the involved tooth, using the adjacent teeth and the spaces between them for retention. Have the patient bite to be sure neither the bands nor the "splint" interferes with bringing the teeth together.
      - Glass ionomer cement can be used as a substitute for IRM. It has the advantage of readily bonding to teeth.
      - If a glass ionomer cement was not used, cover the calcium hydroxide or zinc-eugenol base and adjacent enamel with several coats of cavity varnish (Copalite). Cavity varnish has low solubility in oral fluids.
    - This can provide protection for up to 6 weeks. Have the patient see a dentist as soon as possible.
  - Extensive fractures involving the dentin and exposed pulp
    - Anesthetize the tooth if available and trained to do so.
    - Wash gently with warm saline.
    - Isolate and dry the tooth with cotton gauze or rolls.
    - Cover the pulp and dentin with a mix of calcium hydroxide (Dycal), and allow to harden. Apply several coats of cavity varnish to the calcium hydroxide base.

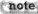

note

Do not use zinc oxide and eugenol to cover the pulp—it causes necrosis of the pulp.

- If a glass ionomer cement is available, it can be substituted for the calcium hydroxide (Dycal). A condensable type of glass ionomer is preferable. Do not coat a glass ionomer cement with cavity varnish.
- The efficiency of this treatment regimen depends on the size of the pulp exposure. If the exposure is larger than 1.5 mm, consider extraction. If all you have available is zinc oxide and eugenol, you must also consider extraction.
- Evacuate for consultant care.

Preserving/Transporting an Avulsed Tooth

If the tooth has been saved, transport the avulsed tooth in any clean, liquid medium (saline, milk, or saliva). Do not let tooth dry out. Gently rinse tooth with 0.9% normal saline. Do not scrape off any debris or attempt to scale the tooth. A completely avulsed tooth may be permanently retained if replaced in the socket with minimal handling in less than one hour.

Temporary Restorations

- Remove as much of the soft decayed material as possible with a spoon-shaped instrument. If the patient is properly anesthetized, he or she should feel no pain.
- Irrigate the cavity with warm water until loose debris has been flushed out.
- Isolate the tooth with gauze packs and gently dry the cavity with cotton pellets.
- Mix the intermediate restorative material (IRM) zinc oxide powder with two or three drops of IRM liquid (eugenol) on a clean dry surface (parchment pad) until a thick putty-like mix is obtained. Adding a drop of water to the mixture will quicken setting.
- Fill the cavity with the IRM putty, tamping it gently (use the Woodson Plastic Instrument no. 2 or no. 3, or a moistened cotton tip applicator).
- Have the patient bite several times to compress the putty and to avoid malocclusion problems with opposite teeth when dry.
- Remove surplus filling material by lightly rubbing the tooth with a moist cotton pellet.

- The pain should disappear in a few minutes, and the putty will harden within 5 to 10 minutes. Caution the patient not to chew on the treated tooth.
- If IRM is not available, a cotton pellet impregnated with eugenol may be left in the cavity. Glass ionomer cement is an excellent substitute for the IRM. A condensable glass ionomer is preferable, but any type will work. Glass ionomer can be placed directly against exposed pulpal tissue.
- Instruct the patient that the procedure is temporary and that a dentist must give definitive care.

Gunshot Wounds/Blast Injuries

Overview

The incidence of blast injuries increases during warfare, but these injuries are also becoming more common in the civilian world as terrorist activities and hazardous material incidents increase. Blasts may injure 70% of the people in the vicinity, whereas automatic weapons used against the same size group may injure only 30%. Mines, shipyards, chemical plants, refineries, fireworks firms, factories, and grain elevators are a particular hazard. However, because many volatile materials are transported by truck or rail, and domestic and bottled gas are common household items, an explosion can occur almost anywhere. An explosion can be divided into three phases: primary, secondary, and tertiary. Different types of injuries occur during these three phases.

- Primary injuries are caused by the pressure wave of the blast. They usually occur in the gas-containing organs, such as the lungs and the gastrointestinal tract. Primary injuries include pulmonary bleeding, pneumothorax, air emboli, or perforation of the gastrointestinal organs. Pressure waves rupture and tear the small vessels and membranes of the gas-containing organs (cavitation) and may also injure the central nervous system. These waves may cause severe damage or death without external signs of injury. Burns occur on unprotected body areas that are facing the source of the explosion.
- Secondary injuries occur when the victim is struck by flying glass, falling mortar, or other debris from the blast. Secondary injuries include lacerations, fractures, and burns.
- Tertiary injuries occur when the victim becomes a missile and is thrown against an object. Injury will occur at the point of impact, and the force of the blast will be transferred to other organs of the body as the energy from the impact is absorbed. Tertiary injuries are usually

apparent, but the prehospital care provider must look for associated injuries according to the type of impact that occurred. The injuries that occur in the tertiary phase are similar to those sustained in ejections from vehicles and falls from significant heights.

Secondary and tertiary injuries are the most obvious and are usually the most aggressively treated. Primary injuries may be the most severe, but they are often overlooked and sometimes never suspected. Adequate assessment of the various kinds of injuries is vital if the prehospital care provider is to manage the patient properly. Blast injuries often cause severe complications that may result in death if they are overlooked or ignored.

Factors Affecting the Frontal Surface Area of Projectiles

The larger the frontal area of a moving missile, the greater the number of particles that will be hit; therefore, the greater the energy exchange that occurs and the larger the cavity that is created. The frontal surface area of the projectile is influenced by three factors: profile, tumble, and fragmentation. Energy exchange or potential energy exchange can be analyzed based on these factors.

○ Profile: An object's initial size and whether that size changes at the time of impact. The profile, or frontal area, of an ice pick is much smaller that that of a baseball bat, which is in turn much smaller than that of a truck. A hollow-pointed missile, if crushed and deformed as a result of striking a body, will have a much larger frontal area than it possessed before its shape was changed. A hollow-point bullet flattens and spreads on impact. This change enlarges the frontal area so that it hits more tissue particles and produces greater energy exchange. A larger cavity forms, and more injury results.

In general, as a bullet travels through the air after being discharged from the weapon, it will strike fewer air particles and maintain most of its speed if its frontal area is kept small and streamlined by its conical shape. If that missile strikes the skin and becomes deformed, covering a larger area, a much greater energy exchange will occur than if its frontal surface area did not expand.

○ Tumble: Whether the object tumbles and assumes a different angle inside the body. A wedge-shaped bullet's center of gravity is located nearer to the base than to the nose of the bullet. When the nose of the bullet strikes something, it slows rapidly. Momentum continues to carry the base of the bullet forward, with the center of gravity seeking to become the leading point of the bullet. This movement causes an end-over-end motion, or tumble. As the bullet tumbles, the normally horizontal sides of the bullet become its leading edge. More energy exchange is produced, and therefore greater tissue damage occurs.

○ Fragmentation: Whether the object breaks up after it enters the body. Bullets such as those with soft noses or vertical cuts in the nose, and safety slugs that contain many small fragments, increase body damage by breaking apart on impact. The mass of fragments produced constitutes a larger frontal area than a single solid bullet, and energy is dispersed rapidly into the tissue. If the missile shatters, it will spread out over a wider area, with two results: (1) More tissue particles will be struck by the larger frontal projection, and (2) the injuries will be distributed over a larger portion of the body because more organs will be struck. The multiple pieces of shot from a shotgun blast produce similar results. Shotgun wounds are an excellent example of the fragmentation injury pattern.

Reprinted from *PHTLS Basic and Advanced Prehospital Trauma Life Support*, Fifth Edition, by National Association of Emergency Medical Technicians. Copyright 2005, with permission from Elsevier.

Entrance and Exit Wounds

Before applying the dressing, carefully examine the casualty to determine if there is more than one wound. A missile may have entered at one point and exited at another point. The exit wound is usually *larger* than the entrance wound.

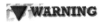 **WARNING**

Casualties should be continually monitored for the development of conditions that may require the performance of necessary basic lifesaving measures, such as clearing the airway and performing mouth-to-mouth resuscitation. All open (or penetrating) wounds should be checked for a point of entry and exit and treated accordingly.

WARNING

If the missile lodges in the body (fails to exit), *do not* attempt to remove it or probe the wound. Apply a dressing. If there is an object extending from (impaled in) the wound, *do not* remove the object. Apply a dressing around the object and use additional improvised bulky materials/dressings (use the cleanest material available) to build up the area around the object. Apply a supporting bandage over the bulky materials to hold them in place.

Considerations for Gunshot Wounds and Blast Injuries

1 Wounding mechanisms
- Blast injury
- Cavitation
- Crush injury
- Embolization
- Fractures
- Laceration
- Perforation

2 Prehospital treatment of penetrating injuries
- Assessment
  - Airway: Special considerations for trauma victims
  - Breathing
    - Pneumothorax
    - Hemothorax
    - Flail chest
    - Pulmonary contusion
  - Circulation
    - Hemorrhage
    - Hypovolemia
    - Cardiac tamponade
    - Embolus
  - Deficits
    - Nerve damage
    - Head injuries
    - Bone and ligament injuries

Head Injury

Performance Steps

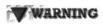 **WARNING**

Treat casualties with any type of traumatic head injury or loss of consciousness as if they have a spinal injury.

1 Take appropriate body substance isolation precautions.

② Check for the signs and symptoms of head injuries.

○ Superficial wound
  ■ Lacerated, torn, ragged, or mangled skin tissue
  ■ Copious bleeding, possible exposed skull

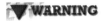 **WARNING**

Do not manipulate the wound to observe the skull.

○ Closed head injury: Caused by a direct blow to the head

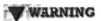 **WARNING**

Brain injury, leading to a loss of function or death, often occurs without evidence of a skull fracture or scalp injury. Because the skull cannot expand, swelling of the brain or a collection of fluid pressing on the brain can cause pressure. This can compress and destroy the brain tissue.

  ■ Deformity of the head
  ■ Clear fluid or blood escaping from the nose and/or ear(s)
  ■ Periorbital discoloration (raccoon eyes)
  ■ Bruising behind the ears, over the mastoid process (battle sign)
  ■ Lowered pulse rate if the casualty has not lost a significant amount of blood
  ■ Signs of increased intracranial pressure
    · Headache, nausea, and/or vomiting
    · Possible unconsciousness
    · Change in pupil size or symmetry
    · Lateral loss of motor nerve function—one side of the body becomes paralyzed

note

Lateral loss may not happen immediately but may occur later.

    · Change in the casualty's respiratory rate or pattern
    · A steady rise in the systolic blood pressure if the casualty has not lost significant amounts of blood (with slower pulse rate)

- A rise in the pulse pressure (systolic pressure minus diastolic pressure)
- Elevated body temperature
- Restlessness: Indicates insufficient oxygenation of the brain
○ Concussion: Caused by a violent jar or shock

 note

A direct blow to the skull may bruise the brain.

- Temporary unconsciousness followed by confusion.
- Temporary, usually short-term, loss of some or all brain functions.
- The casualty has a headache or is seeing double.
- The casualty may or may not have a skull fracture.
○ Contusion: An internal bruise or injury. It is more serious than a concussion. The injured tissue may bleed or swell. Swelling may cause increased intracranial pressure, which may result in a decreased level of consciousness and even death.
○ Open head injury
  - Penetrating wound: An entry wound with no exit wound
  - Perforating wound: Both entry and exit wounds
  - Visibly deformed skull
  - Exposed brain tissue
  - Possible unconsciousness
  - Paralysis or disability on one side of the body
  - Change in pupil size

3 Perform direct manual stabilization of the casualty's head and neck. In the case of penetrating trauma during a combat operation, stabilization of the head and neck is not necessary while under enemy fire.

4 Check the casualty's vital signs.

5 Assess the casualty's level of consciousness using the AVPU scale.

○ A (Alert): The casualty responds spontaneously to stimuli and is able to answer questions in a clear manner.
○ V (Verbal): The casualty does not respond spontaneously but is responsive to verbal stimuli.
○ P (Pain): The casualty does not respond spontaneously or to verbal stimuli but is responsive to painful stimuli.
○ U (Unresponsive): The casualty is unresponsive to any stimuli.

6 Assess the casualty's pupil size.

○ Observe the size of each pupil.

> **note**
>
> A variation of pupil size may indicate a brain injury. In a very small percentage of people, unequal pupil size is normal.

○ Shine a light into each eye to observe the pupillary reaction to light.

> **note**
>
> The pupils should constrict promptly when exposed to bright light. Failure of the pupils to constrict may indicate brain injury.

7 Assess the casualty's motor function.

○ Evaluate the casualty's strength, mobility, coordination, and sensation.
○ Document any complaints, weakness, or numbness.

> **note**
>
> Progressive loss of strength or sensation is an important indicator of brain injury.

8 Treat the head injury.

○ Superficial head injury
  ■ Apply a pressure dressing.
  ■ Observe for abnormal behavior or evidence of complications.
○ Head injury involving deep trauma
  ■ If the patient is unconscious, insert a nasopharyngeal airway without hyperextending the neck.
  ■ Administer high-concentration oxygen by nonrebreather mask and evaluate the need for artificial ventilations with supplemental oxygen (if available).
  ■ Apply a cervical collar.
  ■ Dress the head wound(s).
  ■ Control bleeding.

> **⚠ WARNING**
>
> Do not apply pressure to or replace exposed brain tissue.

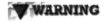

- Treat for shock. (Hypovolemia is a significant cause of morbidity and mortality.)
- Monitor the casualty for convulsions or seizures.
- Position the casualty with the head elevated 6 inches to assist with the drainage of blood from the brain.

> **CAUTION**
> Do not give the casualty anything by mouth.

9 Continue to monitor the casualty and check and record the following at 5-minute intervals.

- Level of consciousness
- Pupillary responsiveness and equality
- Vital signs
- Motor functions

10 Record the treatment on the appropriate form.

11 Evacuate the casualty.

Heat Injury

Performance Steps

1 Identify the type of heat injury based upon the following characteristic signs and symptoms.

- Heat cramps—muscle cramps of the arms, legs, and/or abdomen
- Heat exhaustion
  - Often
    - Profuse sweating and pale (or gray), moist, cool skin
    - Headache
    - Weakness or faintness
    - Dizziness
    - Loss of appetite or nausea
  - Sometimes
    - Heat cramps
    - Nausea (with or without vomiting)
    - Urge to defecate
    - Chills

- Rapid breathing
- Tingling sensation of the hands and feet
- Confusion

○ Heat stroke
  - Rapid onset, with the core body temperature rising to above 106°F (41°C) within 10 to 15 minutes
  - Hot, dry skin
  - Headache
  - Dizziness
  - Nausea (stomach pains)
  - Confusion
  - Weakness
  - Loss of consciousness
  - Possible seizures
  - Weak and rapid pulse and respirations

② Provide the proper first aid for the heat injury.

○ Heat cramps
  - Move the casualty to a cool shaded area, if possible.
  - Loosen the casualty's clothing unless he or she is in a chemical environment.
  - Give the casualty at least one canteen of oral hydration solution (dissolve 1 packet in a canteen of water). If oral hydration solution is unavailable, give plain water.
  - Evacuate the casualty if the cramps are not relieved after treatment.

○ Heat exhaustion
  - Conscious casualty
    - Move the casualty to a shaded area, if possible.
    - Loosen and/or remove the casualty's clothing and boots unless he or she is in a chemical environment.
    - Pour water on the casualty and fan him or her, if possible.
    - Slowly give the casualty one canteen of oral hydration solution.
    - Elevate the casualty's legs.
  - An unconscious casualty or one who is nauseated, unable to retain fluids, or whose symptoms have not improved after 20 minutes
    - Cool the casualty as discussed earlier.
    - Evacuate the casualty to an MTF for IV therapy or, if qualified, initiate an IV infusion of Ringer's lactate or sodium chloride.

○ Heat stroke

CAUTION

Heat stroke is a medical emergency. If the casualty is not cooled rapidly, the body cells, especially the brain cells, are literally cooked; irreversible damage is done to the central nervous system. The casualty must be evacuated to the nearest medical treatment facility immediately.

- Conscious casualty
  - Remove the casualty's outer garments and/or protective clothing, if possible.
  - Keep the casualty out of the direct sun, if possible.
  - Immerse the casualty in cold water, if available, and massage him or her.

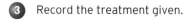 **WARNING**

Cooling with cold water immersion may produce shivering, increasing the core temperature.

  - Lay the casualty down and elevate his or her legs.
  - Have the casualty slowly drink at least one canteen of oral hydration solution.
  - Evacuate the casualty to an MTF for IV therapy or, if qualified, initiate an IV infusion of Ringer's lactate or sodium chloride to maintain a systolic blood pressure of at least 90 mm Hg.
- Unconscious casualty or one who is vomiting or unable to retain oral fluids
  - Cool the casualty as discussed previously but give nothing by mouth.
  - Initiate an IV, if qualified.
  - Evacuate the casualty.

3 Record the treatment given.

Hemorrhage Control Guidelines
Overview

Hemorrhage continues to be a leading cause of death on the battlefield. In Vietnam more than 2,500 deaths were attributed to hemorrhage in patients who had only extremity wounds. There is a new philosophy on controlling hemorrhage through the initial use of tourniquets in addition to the old standbys of direct pressure, pressure dressings, pressure points, and elevation. In addition, there is a new hemostatic agent available, which has proven effective in controlling moderate to severe hemorrhage.

Product

QuikClot is a dehydrated granular powder marketed by Z-Medica. It has been shown to rapidly control moderate to severe bleeding in animal models. There is some concern that an exothermic reaction created by the powder can damage surrounding tissue when not used in accordance with the manufacturer's directions. QuikClot is recommended only for use with external wounds.

Directions

The primary means of controlling severe hemorrhage while under direct enemy fire will continue to be the initial use of an effective tourniquet. Once the tactical situation allows, conventional means to control hemorrhage, such as direct pressure, pressure dressings, pressure points, or elevation, should be employed. If conventional methods are ineffective in controlling hemorrhage, then use of the QuikClot hemostatic agent would be appropriate.

1. Blot away excess blood, water, and dirt from the wound with a sterile gauze pad or the cleanest, driest product available.

2. Tear open the QuikClot pack, holding it away from your and the patient's face. (Avoid breathing the dust from QuikClot because it may irritate the eyes, nose, throat, and skin: Burns can result.)

3. Apply contents of bag directly into the wound. Use only a sufficient amount to stop the bleeding.

4. Apply direct firm pressure to the wound using a sterile gauze bandage or the cleanest product available. Hold for several minutes.

5. Wrap and tie a bandage so as to maintain pressure on the wound.

6. Evacuate the patient as soon as possible.

7. Send empty package along with the patient.

8. Discard unused portion after opening.

note

Prior to irrigation, attending medical personnel should brush away all loose granules of QuikClot. Flood the entire area with irrigation solution, then proceed with normal irrigation and/or aspiration until you have removed all visible granules.

▼ **WARNING**

QuikClot should *not* be poured into internal cavities (abdominal, thoracic, or cranial) in an attempt to stop internal bleeding. QuikClot is for external bleeding only.

note

QuikClot may be affected by rain prior to or during use.

Summary

Battlefield hemorrhage continues to be the leading cause of preventable death in combat. In the event you are unable to control hemorrhage with conventional methods, QuikClot may be an adjunct in hemorrhage control that can save soldiers' lives.

High-Altitude Illness

Performance Steps

1. Understand the physics involved with high-altitude illness.

○ Atmospheric pressure decreases as altitude increases.
○ The percentage of oxygen in the atmosphere remains constant.
○ The result is that the partial pressure of oxygen decreases with altitude.
○ At 18,000 feet, the partial pressure of oxygen is about half that at sea level.

2. Recognize the signs and symptoms of various types of high-altitude illness.

○ Acute mountain sickness (AMS)

note

AMS is the most common form of altitude sickness and may develop at altitudes as low as 6,500 feet.

- Headache.
- Fatigue.
- Nausea.
- Dyspnea.
- Sleep disturbances.
- Symptoms are aggravated by exertion.

note

AMS may evolve into high-altitude pulmonary edema, high-altitude cerebral edema, or both.

○ High-altitude cerebral edema (HACE)

note

HACE is believed to be present to a mild degree in all forms of altitude sickness.

- Gait ataxia is a reliable early warning sign.
- Headache.
- Mental confusion.
- Hallucinations.
- Stiff neck does not occur.

▼ **WARNING**

Coma and death may develop within a few hours of the first warning signs of HACE.

○ High-altitude pulmonary edema (HAPE)

note

HAPE usually develops 24 to 96 hours after rapid ascent above 8,000 feet.

- HAPE is characterized by increasing dyspnea.
- Irritative cough produces frothy, often bloody sputum.

- Weakness.
- Cyanosis.
- Low-grade fever.
- Tachycardia.
- Fine or coarse rales.
- Coma.

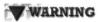

> **WARNING**
>
> HAPE may worsen rapidly. Coma and death may occur within hours.

---

3 Initiate prophylactic measures to prevent high-altitude illnesses.

○ Altitude sickness is best prevented by slow ascent.
- Most individuals can ascend to 5,000 feet in 1 day without symptoms.
- Above 5,000 feet, a rate of 1,500 feet per day is advisable.

> **note** ————————————————————————
>
> All rates are variable. A climber should learn how fast he or she can ascend without developing symptoms. A climbing party should be paced to its slowest member.

○ Although physical fitness enables greater exertion with lower oxygen consumption, it does not protect against any form of altitude sickness.
○ Increased hydration with moderate salt restriction may prevent or diminish symptoms of AMS.
○ Eating frequent, small meals that are high in easily digestible carbohydrates improves altitude tolerance.
○ Acetazolamide (Diamox) 125 mg at bedtime or 125 mg every 8 hours for susceptible persons is an effective prophylactic for AMS. It should be started on the first day that the patient is at high altitude.

4 Manage high-altitude illnesses.

○ AMS
- Increase fluid intake.
- Give aspirin or a nonsteroidal anti-inflammatory drug (NSAID) for altitude headache.
- Administer an antiemetic.
- Keep patient on a light diet.

- Restrict activity.
- Descend, if symptoms worsen or are intractable.
○ HACE
  - HACE requires immediate descent. Pressurization in a hyperbaric bag may buy time if descent is not possible.
  - Acetazolamide (Diamox) 125-250 mg twice a day.
  - Dexamethasone 4 mg PO, IM, or IV every 6 hours.
○ HAPE
  - Bedrest and oxygen at high altitude may be tried with mild HAPE, depending on mission requirements.
  - If the condition worsens, immediate descent is essential.

---

note

On the basis of mission parameters, a portable hyperbaric bag may be transported and used as a temporary substitute for descent. However, this will only buy time for mission completion, and descent must be accomplished at the earliest opportunity.

  - Once descent is accomplished, the patient should be continued on oxygen and managed as one would with other forms of pulmonary edema.
  - When promptly treated, patients usually recover from HAPE within 24 to 48 hours after descent.

Hypothermia

Performance Steps

1 Recognize the signs and symptoms of hypothermia.

○ Generalized hypothermia is caused by prolonged exposure to low temperatures, especially with wind and wet conditions, and it may be caused by immersion in cold water.

CAUTION

With generalized hypothermia, the entire body has cooled, with the core temperature below 95°F (35°C). This is a medical emergency.

  - Moderate hypothermia

Moderate hypothermia should be suspected in any chronically ill person who is found in an environment of less than 50°F (10°C).

- Conscious, but usually apathetic or lethargic
- Shivering, with pale, cold skin; slurred speech; poor muscle coordination; faint pulse
■ Severe hypothermia
  - Unconscious or stuporous
  - Ice cold skin
  - Inaudible heart beat or irregular heart rhythm
  - Unobtainable blood pressure
  - Unreactive pupils
  - Very slow respirations

2 Treat the hypothermia.
○ Generalized hypothermia
  ■ Moderate hypothermia
    - Remove the casualty from the cold environment.
    - Replace wet clothing with dry clothing.
    - Cover the casualty with insulating material or blankets.
    - If available, apply heating pads to the casualty's armpits, groin, and abdomen.

If far from a medical treatment facility and if the situation and facilities permit, immerse the casualty in a tub of 104°F (40°C) water; keep extremities out of the water, allowing the central core to warm first. This is a last-ditch method for warming; every attempt should be made to evacuate the casualty.

- If available, slowly give sugar and sweet, warm fluids.

CAUTION

Do not give the casualty alcohol.

- Wrap the casualty from head to toe.
- Evacuate the casualty lying down.

■ Severe hypothermia

Handle the casualty very gently.

- Cut away wet clothing and replace it with dry clothing.
- Maintain the airway.
  - Administer oxygen if trained personnel and equipment are available.
  - Assist with ventilation if the casualty's respiration rate is less than 5 breaths per minute.

note

Do not use artificial airways or suctioning devices.

Do not hyperventilate the casualty. Keep the rate of artificial ventilation at approximately 8 to 10 breaths per minute.

- Monitor the patient's pulse. If none is detected, apply automatic external defibrillator, if available. Begin CPR. IV fluids should be warmed to 104°F (40°C) before administration.
- Handle the casualty gently; rough handling can precipitate cardiac arrhythmias.

note

The treatment of moderate hypothermia is aimed at preventing further heat loss and rewarming the casualty as rapidly as possible. Rewarming a casualty with severe hypothermia is critical to saving his or her life, but the kind of care that rewarming requires is nearly impossible to carry out in the field. Evacuate the casualty promptly to a medical treatment facility. Use stabilizing measures en route.

Immunizations

Table 2 provides an overview of required immunizations.

note

If a series has been started, and the time since the last dose is greater than the recommended interval for administration of the next dose, *do not restart the series;* give the next dose and inform the patient when he or she must return for the remainder of the series, if additional doses are required.

Table 2	Required Immunizations		
Vaccine	**Initial Dosage and Route**	**Booster Dose**	**Comments**
Anthrax	0.5 mL SC at 0, 2, and 4 weeks, then at 6, 12, and 18 months	0.5 mL SC annually	Annual booster
Hepatitis A	1.0 mL IM at 0 and 6-12 months (Havrix or VAQTA)	None currently required	——
Hepatitis B	1.0 mL IM at 0, 1, and 6 months	None currently required	——
Influenza	0.5 mL IM annually in October	0.5 mL IM at 6 months if still in risk area	Annual; consider booster if in southern hemisphere during April to September
Japanese B encephalitis	1.0 mL SC at 0, 7, and 30 days	1.0 mL SC every 3 years	By geographic area only
Measles	0.5 mL SC of Attenuvax or MMR (preferred)	None currently required	Required if no serologic evidence of previous exposure
Meningococcal	0.5 mL SC single dose	0.5 mL SC every 5 years	More frequent boosters for some countries
Mumps	0.5 mL SC of Mumpsvax or MMR (preferred)	None currently required	Required if no serologic evidence of previous exposure
Plague	Two of three-shot series, 1.0 mL IM at 0 months, then 0.2 mL at 1-3 months	0.2 mL IM upon deployment to a risk area and every 6 months while there	Boost at direction of unit surgeon for high-risk areas (CDC blue sheet)
Polio	IPV (inactivated polio vaccine), 0.5 mL SC at 0, 1-2, and 6-12 months.	0.5 mL SC for travel to highly endemic areas	Boost at direction of unit surgeon for high-risk areas
Rabies	0.1 mL ID (or 1.0 mL IM) at 0, 7, and 21-28 days. Do not mix ID and IM doses within a series. Must use IM dosing if taking chloroquine or mefloquine within 14 days of any dose.	None currently required	Initial series for personnel in medical SOF and for personnel assigned, attached, or OPCON to an operational team

Vaccine	Initial Dosage and Route	Booster Dose	Comments
Rubella	0.5 mL SC of MMR (preferred) or Meruvax II	None currently required	Required if no serologic evidence of previous exposure
Tetanus-diphtheria toxoid (absorbed)	0.5 mL IM at 0, 1-2, and 8-14 months	0.5 mL IM every 10 years or as prophylaxis after severe/dirty wounds	Required if no documentation of previous immunization
Typhoid (two types of vaccine used)	a) Injectable vaccine (Typhim Vi [Pasteur-Mérieux Connaught]): 0.5 mL IM b) Oral vaccine (Vivotif Berna [Berna]): One capsule every other day for a total of four capsules	a) Boost with same vaccine if possible. Typhim Vi 0.5 mL IM every 2 years b) Berna oral vaccine: Repeat four-dose series every 5 years.	For capsules, do not lengthen interval. Swallow (do not chew) with cool drink 1 hr before a meal. Do not take within 24 hours of taking mefloquine or antibiotics.
Varicella	0.5 mL SC at 0 and 1-2 months	None currently required	Required if no serologic evidence of previous exposure
Yellow fever	0.5 mL SC	0.5 mL SC every 10 years	None
Smallpox	3 pricks with bifurcated needle	15 pricks with bifurcated needle every 10 years	Check with CDC for continued requirement

CDC, Centers of Disease Control and Prevention; ID, intradermal; IM, intramuscular; MMR, measles-mumps-rubella; OPCON, operational control; SC, subcutaneous; SOF, special operations forces.

note

Multiple live virus vaccines may be given the same day. *If they are not given the same day*, they must be separated by 30 days. Live virus vaccines are as follows: oral polio, yellow fever, measles, mumps, rubella, and adenovirus.

note

Only three inactivated vaccines are given at one time and at separate sites. Only one inactivated and one live virus (MMR, yellow fever, smallpox) may be given on the same day.

Mental Health

Overview

During actual combat, military operations continue around the clock at a constant pace, often under severe weather conditions. Terrible things happen in combat. During such periods the soldier's mental and physical endurance will be pushed to the limit. Psychological first aid will help sustain the soldier's mental and physical performance during normal activities, and especially during military operations under extremely adverse conditions and in hostile environments.

Battle Fatigue and Other Combat Stress Reactions

Battle fatigue is a temporary emotional disorder or inability to function experienced by a previously normal soldier as a reaction to the over-whelming or cumulative stress of combat. By definition, battle fatigue gets better with reassurance, rest, physical replenishment, and activities that restore confidence. Physical fatigue, or sleep loss, although commonly present, is not necessary for a diagnosis of battle fatigue. All combat and combat support troops are likely to feel battle fatigue under conditions of intense and/or prolonged stress. They may even become battle fatigue casualties, unable to perform their mission roles for hours or days.

Other negative behaviors may be combat stress reactions (CSRs), but are not called battle fatigue because they require treatment other than simple rest, replenishment, and restoration of confidence. These negative CSRs include drug and alcohol abuse, committing atrocities against enemy prisoners and noncombatants, looting, desertion, and self-inflicted wounds. These harmful CSRs can often be prevented by good psychological first aid; however, if these negative actions occur, these persons may require disciplinary action instead of reassurance and rest.

Reactions to Stress

Most people react to misfortune or disasters (military or civilian, threatened or actual) after the situation has passed. All people feel some fear. This fear may be greater than they have experienced at any other time or they may be more aware of their fear. In such a situation, they should not be surprised if they feel shaky and/or become sweaty, nauseated, or confused. These reactions are normal and are not a cause for concern. However, some reactions, either short or long term, will cause problems if left unchecked. The following disorders are consequences of too much stress.

○ Emotional reactions
  ■ The most common stress reactions are simply inefficient perform-ances, such as the following:
    • Slow thinking (or reaction time).
    • Difficulty sorting out the important things from all the noise and seeing what needs to be done.
    • Difficulty getting started.
    • Indecisiveness, trouble focusing attention.
    • A tendency to do familiar tasks and be preoccupied with familiar details. This can reach the point where the person is very passive, such as just sitting or wandering about not knowing what to do.
  ■ Much less common reactions to a disaster or accident may be uncontrolled emotional outbursts, such as crying, screaming, or laughing. Some soldiers will react in the opposite way. They will be very withdrawn and silent and try to isolate themselves from everyone. These soldiers should be encouraged to remain with their assigned unit. Uncontrolled reactions may appear by them-selves or in any combination (the soldier may be crying uncontrol-lably one minute and then laughing the next or may lie down and babble like a child). In this state, the soldier is restless and cannot keep still. He or she may run about, apparently without purpose. Inside, the soldier feels great rage or fear, and his or her physical acts may show this. In his or her anger, the individual may indis-criminately strike out at others.

○ Loss of adaptability
  ■ In a desperate attempt to get away from the danger that has over-whelmed them, soldiers may panic and become confused. In the midst of a mortar attack, they may suddenly lose the ability to hear or see. A soldier's mental ability may be so impaired that he or she cannot think clearly or even follow simple commands. Soldiers may stand up in the midst of enemy fire or rush into a burning building because their judgment is clouded and they cannot understand the likely consequences of their behavior. They may lose the ability to move (freezing) and may seem paralyzed. The soldier may faint.
  ■ In other cases, overwhelming stress may produce symptoms that are often associated with head injuries. For example, the soldier may appear dazed or be found wandering around aimlessly. He or she may appear confused and disoriented and may seem to have a complete or partial loss of memory. In such cases, especially when

no eyewitnesses can provide evidence that the person has *not* suffered a head injury, it is necessary for medical personnel to provide rapid evaluation for that possibility.

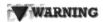 **WARNING**

In cases of possible head injury, do not allow soldiers to expose themselves to further personal danger until the cause of the problem has been determined.

○ Sleep disturbance and repetitions
  ■ A person who has been overwhelmed by disaster or some other stress often has difficulty sleeping. The soldier may experience nightmares related to the disaster, such as dreaming that his or her spouse, parents, or other important people in the soldier's life were killed in the disaster. Remember that nightmares, in themselves, are not considered abnormal when they occur soon after a period of intensive combat or disaster. As time passes, the nightmares usually become less frequent and less intense.
  ■ In extreme cases, a soldier, even when awake, may think repeatedly of the disaster, feel as though it is happening again, and act out parts of his or her stress over and over again. For some persons, this repetitious re-experiencing of the stressful event may be necessary for eventual recovery; therefore, it should not be discouraged or viewed as abnormal. For the person re-experiencing the event, such a reaction may be disruptive and disturbing regardless of the reassurance given to the individual that it is perfectly normal. In such a situation, a short cut that is often possible involves getting the person to talk extensively, even repetitiously, about the experience or his or her feelings. This should not be forced; rather, the soldier should be given repeated opportunities and supportive encouragement to talk in private, preferably to one person. This process is known as "ventilation."

Other Factors

In studies of sudden civilian disasters, a rule of thumb is that 70% to 80% of people will fall into the first category (i.e., emotional reactions). Ten percent to 15% will show the more severe disturbances (i.e., loss of adaptability, sleep disturbances, and/or repetitions). Another 10% to 15% will work effectively and coolly. The latter usually have had prior experience in disasters or have jobs that can be applied effectively in the disaster situation. Military training, like the training of police, fire, and emergency medical specialists in the civilian sector, is designed to shift the proportions so that 99% to 100% of the unit works effectively. But sudden, unexpected horrors, combined with physical fatigue, exhaustion, and distracting worries about the home front, can sometimes throw even well-trained individuals for a temporary loss.

Psychiatric Complications

Although the behaviors described previously usually diminish with time, some do not. A person who has not improved somewhat within a day, even though he or she has been given warm food, time for sleep, and opportunity to ventilate, or who becomes worse, deserves specialized medical/psychiatric care. Do not wait to see if what the soldier is experiencing will get better with time.

Severe Stress or Battle Fatigue Reactions

You do not need specialized training to recognize severe stress or battle fatigue reactions that will cause problems to the soldier, the unit, or the mission. Reactions that are less severe, however, are more difficult to detect. To determine whether a person needs help, you must observe the individual to see whether he or she is doing something meaningful, performing his or her duties, taking care of himself or herself, or behaving in an unusual fashion or acting out of character.

Application of Psychological First Aid

Emotionally disturbed soldiers have built barriers against fear. Soldiers do this for their own protection, although they are probably not aware of doing it. If soldiers find that they do not have to be afraid and that there are normal, understandable things around them, the soldiers will feel safer in dropping these barriers. Persistent efforts to make soldiers realize that you want to understand them will be reassuring, especially if you remain calm. Nothing can cause an emotionally disturbed person to become even more fearful than feeling that others are afraid of him or her. Try to remain calm. Familiar things, such as a cup of coffee, the use of the soldier's name, attention to a minor wound, being given a simple job to do, or the sight of familiar people and activities will add to the soldier's ability to overcome his or her fear. The soldier may not respond well if you get excited, angry, or abrupt.

o Ventilation: After the soldier becomes calmer, he or she is likely to have dreams about the stressful event. The individual also may think about it when awake or even repeat his or her personal reaction to the event. One benefit of this natural pattern is that it helps the soldier master the stress by going over it, just as one masters the initial fear of jumping from a diving board by doing it over and over again. Eventually, it is difficult to remember how frightening the event was initially. In giving first aid to emotionally disturbed soldiers, you should let them follow this natural pattern. Encourage the soldier to talk. Be a good listener. Let the soldier tell, in his or her own words, what actually happened (or what he or she thinks happened). If home front problems or worries have contributed to the stress, it will help soldiers to talk about them. Your patient listening will prove that you are interested in them, and by describing their personal catastrophes, soldiers can work at mastering their fear.

If a soldier becomes overwhelmed in the telling, suggest a cup of coffee or a break. Whatever you do, assure him or her that you will listen again as soon as he or she is ready. Do try to help put the soldier's perception of what happened back into realistic perspective; but *do not* argue about it. For example, if a soldier feels guilty for surviving while his or her teammates were all killed, reassure the soldier that they would be glad he or she is still alive and that others in the unit need him or her now. If the soldier feels responsible for their deaths because of some oversight or mistake (which may be true), a nonpunishing, nonaccusing attitude may help him or her realize that accidents and mistakes do happen in the confusion of war, but that life, the unit, and the mission must go on. (These same principles apply in civilian disaster settings as well.) With this psychological first aid measure, most soldiers start toward recovery quickly.

○ Activity
  ■ A person who is emotionally disturbed as the result of combat action or a catastrophe is basically a casualty of anxiety and fear. The individual is disabled because he or she has become temporarily overwhelmed by anxiety. A good way to control fear is through activity. Almost all soldiers, for example, experience a considerable sense of anxiety and fear while they are awaiting the opening of a big offensive; this is normally relieved, however, once they begin to move into action. They take pride in effective performance and pleasure in knowing that they are good soldiers, perhaps being completely unaware that overcoming their initial fear was their first major accomplishment.
  ■ Useful activity is very beneficial to emotionally disturbed soldiers who are not physically incapacitated. After you help soldiers get over their initial fear, help them to regain some self-confidence. Make them realize that their job is continuing by finding the soldiers

something useful to do. Encourage these soldiers to be active. Get them to carry litters (but not the severely injured), help load trucks, clean up debris, dig foxholes, or assist with refugees. If possible, get soldiers back to their usual duties. Seek out the individual's strong points and help him or her apply them. Avoid having the soldier just sit around. You may have to provide direction by telling soldiers what to do and where to do it. The instructions should be clear and simple, they should be repeated, and they should be reasonable and obviously possible.

People who have panicked are likely to argue. Respect their feelings, but point out more immediate, obtainable, and demanding needs. Channel their excessive energy and, above all, *do not* argue. If you cannot get a soldier interested in doing more profitable work, it may be necessary to enlist aid in controlling his or her overactivity before it spreads to the group and results in more panic. Prevent the spread of such infectious feelings by restraining and segregating soldiers if necessary.

- Involvement in activity helps soldiers in three ways:
  - They forget themselves.
  - They have an outlet for their excessive tensions.
  - They prove to themselves that they can do something useful. It is amazing how effective this is in helping a person overcome feelings of fear, ineffectiveness, and uselessness.

○ Rest: There are times, particularly in combat, when physical exhaustion is a principal cause for emotional reactions. For the weary, dirty soldier, adequate rest, good water to drink, warm food, and a change of clothes with an opportunity to bathe or shave may provide spectacular results.

○ Group activity: You have probably already noticed that people work, face danger, and handle serious problems better if they are members of a closely knit group. Each individual in such a group supports the other members of the group. For example, you see group spirit in football teams and in school fraternities. Because the individuals share the same interests, goals, and problems, they do more and better work; furthermore, they are less worried because everyone is helping. It is this group spirit that wins games or takes a strategic hill in battle. It is so powerful that it is one of the most effective tools you have in your psychological first aid bag. Getting the emotionally distressed soldier back into the group and letting him or her see its orderly and effective activity will reestablish the soldier's sense of belonging and security and will go far toward making him or her a useful member of the unit.

Reactions and Limitations

○ Up to this point the discussion has been primarily about the feelings of emotionally distressed soldiers. What about your feelings toward them? Whatever the situation, you will have emotional reactions (conscious or unconscious) toward these soldiers. Your reactions can either help or hinder your ability to help them. When you are tired or worried, you may very easily become impatient with a person who is unusually slow or who exaggerates. You may even feel resentful toward such a person. At times when many physically wounded casualties lie about you, it will be especially natural for you to resent disabilities that you cannot see. Physical wounds can be seen and easily accepted. Emotional reactions are more difficult to accept as injuries.

On the other hand, you may tend to be overly sympathetic. Excessive sympathy for incapacitated people can be as harmful as negative feelings in your relationship with them. Distressed soldiers need strong help, but not your sorrow. To overwhelm them with pity will make them feel even more inadequate. You must expect the soldier to recover, be able to return to duty, and become a useful soldier. This expectation should be displayed in your behavior and attitude as well as in what you say. If a soldier can see your calmness, confidence, and competence, he or she will be reassured and will feel a sense of greater security.

○ You may feel guilty at encouraging soldiers to recover and return to an extremely dangerous situation, especially if you are to stay in a safer, more comfortable place. Remember, though, that if they return to duty and do well, they will feel strong and whole. On the other hand, if they are sent home as "psychos," they may have self-doubts and often disabling symptoms the rest of their lives. Another thing to remind yourself is that in combat, someone must fight in such a soldier's place. The temporarily battle fatigued soldier, if he or she returns to his unit and comrades, will be less likely to overload again (or be wounded or killed) than will a new replacement.

○ Above all, you must guard against becoming impatient, intolerant, and resentful, on the one hand, and overly solicitous on the other. Remember that such emotion will rarely help soldiers and can never increase your ability to make clear decisions.

○ As with physically injured soldiers, medical personnel will take over the care of emotionally distressed soldiers who need this specific care as soon as possible. The first aid that they have received from you will be of great value to their recovery.

- Remember that every soldier (even you) has a potential emotional overload point, which varies from individual to individual, from time to time, and from situation to situation. Because a soldier has reacted abnormally to stress in the past does not necessarily mean he or she will react the same way to the next stressful situation. Remember, any soldier, as tough as he or she may seem, is capable of showing signs of anxiety and stress. No one is absolutely immune.

Mild Battle Fatigue

- Physical signs*
  - Trembling, tearful
  - Jumpy, nervous
  - Cold sweat, dry mouth
  - Pounding heart, dizziness
  - Nausea, vomiting, diarrhea
  - Fatigue
  - "Thousand-yard stare"
- Emotional signs*
  - Anxious, indecisive
  - Irritable, complaining
  - Forgetful, unable to concentrate
  - Insomnia, nightmares
  - Easily startled by noises, movement
  - Grief, tearfulness
  - Anger, beginning to lose confidence in self and unit
  - Difficulty thinking, speaking, and communicating
- Self- and buddy-aid
  - Continue mission performance; focus on immediate mission.
  - Expect soldier to perform assigned duties.
  - Remain calm at all times; be directive and in control.
  - Let soldier know his or her reaction is normal, and that there is nothing seriously wrong with the soldier.
  - Keep soldier informed of the situation, objectives, expectations, and support. Control rumors.
  - Build soldier's confidence; talk about succeeding.
  - Keep soldier productive (when not resting) through recreational activities or equipment maintenance.
  - Ensure that soldier maintains good personal hygiene.
  - Ensure that soldier eats, drinks, and sleeps as soon as possible.

---

*Most or all of these signs are present in mild battle fatigue. They can be present in normal soldiers in combat without affecting their ability to do their jobs.

- Let soldier talk about his or her feelings. *Do not* "put down" the soldier's feelings of grief or worry.
- Give practical advice and put emotions into perspective.

More Serious Battle Fatigue

- Physical signs[†]
  - Constantly moves around
  - Flinching or ducking at sudden sounds and movement
  - Shaking, trembling (whole body or arms)
  - Cannot use part of body (e.g., hand, arm, legs), for no physical reason
  - Cannot see, hear, or feel (partial or complete loss)
  - Physical exhaustion, crying
  - Freezing under fire, or total immobility
  - Vacant stares; staggers, sways when stands
  - Panic running under fire
- Emotional signs[†]
  - Rapid and/or inappropriate talking
  - Argumentative, reckless actions
  - Inattentive to personal hygiene
  - Indifferent to danger
  - Memory loss
  - Severe stuttering, mumbling, or inability to speak at all
  - Insomnia, nightmares
  - Seeing or hearing things that do not exist
  - Rapid emotional shifts
  - Social withdrawal
  - Apathy
  - Hysterical outbursts
  - Frantic or strange behavior
- Treatment procedures[‡]
  - If soldier's behavior endangers the mission, self or others, do whatever necessary to control soldier.
  - If soldier is upset, calmly talk him or her into cooperating.
  - If concerned about soldier's reliability:
    - Unload soldier's weapon.
    - Take weapon if seriously concerned.
    - Physically restrain soldier only when necessary for safety or transportation.

[†]These signs are present in addition to the signs of mild battle fatigue reaction.
[‡]Do these procedures in addition to the self- and buddy-aid care.

- Reassure everyone that the signs are probably just battle fatigue and will quickly improve.
- If battle fatigue signs continue:
  - Get soldier to a safer place.
  - *Do not* leave soldier alone; keep someone the soldier knows with him or her.
  - Notify senior NCO or officer.
  - Have soldier examined by medical personnel.
- Give soldier tasks to do when not sleeping, eating, or resting.
- Assure soldier he or she will return to full duty in 24 hours; return soldier to normal duties as soon as he or she is ready.

Preventive Measures to Combat Battle Fatigue

○ Welcome new members into your team and get to know them quickly. If you are new, be active in making friends.
○ Be physically fit (strength, endurance, and agility).
○ Know and practice life-saving self- and buddy-aid.
○ Practice rapid relaxation techniques (FM 26-2).
○ Help each other out when things are tough at home or in the unit.
○ Keep informed; ask your leader questions, and ignore rumors.
○ Work together to give everyone food, water, shelter, hygiene, and sanitation.
○ Sleep when mission and safety permit; let everyone get time to sleep.
  - Sleep only in safe places and by standard operating procedure.
  - If possible, sleep 6 to 9 hours per day.
  - Try to get at least 4 hours sleep per day.
  - Get good sleep before going on sustained operations.
  - Catnap when you can, but allow time to wake up fully.
  - Catch up on sleep after going without.

Spinal Injury

Performance Steps

 Check for the signs and symptoms of a spinal injury.

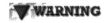

If you suspect that the casualty has a spinal injury, treat the casualty as though he or she does have a spinal injury.

○ Spinal deformity: Its presence indicates a severe spinal injury, but its absence does not rule one out.
○ Tenderness and/or pain in the spinal region.
  ■ Detect it by palpation or ask the casualty.
  ■ The presence of any pain is sufficient cause to suspect the presence of a spinal injury.
○ Lacerations and/or contusions in the spinal region indicate severe trauma and usually accompany a spinal injury.

> **note** ───────────────────────────────
>
> The absence of lacerations and/or contusions does not rule out a spinal injury.

○ Weakness, loss of sensation, and/or paralysis.
  ■ A neck-level (cervical) spine injury may cause numbness or paralysis in all four extremities.
  ■ A waist-level spinal injury may cause numbness or paralysis below the waist.
  ■ Ask the casualty to try to move his or her fingers and toes to check for paralysis.
○ Palpate the spine for tenderness.
  ■ Carefully insert the hand under the neck and feel along the cervical spine as far as can be done without disturbing the casualty's spine.
  ■ Carefully insert the hand into the cavity formed by the small of the back and feel along the thoracic spine and down the lumbar spine as far as possible without disturbing the spine.
  ■ If the casualty says that an area of the spine is tender, consider that he or she has a spinal injury.

❷ Secure the casualty to a short backboard. (If using a Kendrick Extrication Device [KED], go to step 3.)

> **note** ───────────────────────────────
>
> Apply a short backboard when extricating a casualty from a vehicle or location that will not accommodate the use of a long backboard. If available, use a KED, which is a commercial backboard.

- Direct an assistant to immobilize the casualty's head and neck using manual stabilization.
  - Grasp each of the patient's shoulders, one with each hand.
  - Gently position the patient's head between your forearms.
  - Maintain manual stabilization until directed to release the stabilization.
- Apply a cervical collar, if available, or improvise one.
- Push the board as far into the area behind the casualty as possible.
- Tilt the upper end of the board toward the head.
- Direct the assistant to position the back of the casualty's head against the board, maintaining manual stabilization by moving the head and neck as one unit.

> **note**
>
> If the cervical collar or improvised collar does not fit flush with the backboard, place a roll in the hollow space between the neck and board. The roll should only be large enough to fill the gap, not to exert pressure on the neck.

- Secure the casualty's head and head supports to the board with straps or cravats.

> **▼ WARNING**
>
> Ensure that the cravats or head straps are firmly in place before the assistant releases stabilization.

  - Apply head supports.
  - Use two rolled towels, blankets, sandbags, or similar material.
  - Place one close to each side of the head.
  - Using a cravat-like material across the forehead, make the supports and head one unit by tying to the board.
- Secure the casualty to the short backboard.
  - Place the buckle of the first strap in the casualty's lap.
  - Pass the other end of the strap through the lower hole in the board, up the back of the board, through the top hole, under the armpit, over the shoulder, and across the back of the board at the neck.
  - Buckle the second strap to the first strap and place the buckle on the side of the board at the neck.
  - Pass the other end over the shoulder, under the armpit, through the top hole in the board, down the back of the board, through the lower hole, and across the lap. Secure it by buckling it to the first strap.

○ Tie the casualty's hands together and place them in his or her lap.

> **note** ———————————————————————
>
> When positioning a casualty who is secured to a short
> backboard onto a long backboard, line up the hand grip
> holes of the short backboard with the holes of the long
> backboard, if possible, and secure the two boards together.

③ Secure the casualty to a KED.

○ Direct an assistant to immobilize the casualty's head and neck using manual stabilization.
  ■ Rest arms on each of the patient's shoulders, and place the hands on both sides of the casualty's skull, with the palms over the ears.
  ■ Support the jaw (mandible) with the fingers.
  ■ Maintain manual stabilization until directed to release the stabilization.
○ Position the immobilization device behind the patient.
○ Secure the device to the patient's torso.
  ■ Immobilize the torso, from the top to the bottom strap.
  ■ Apply the pelvic straps, ensuring to pad the groin area.
○ Secure the patient's head to the device.
  ■ Pad behind the patient's head as necessary.
  ■ Place one cravat across the chin angle toward the ear, ensuring the cravat does not interfere with the airway. Tie cravats to the side of the device.
  ■ Place a cravat across the forehead angle toward the base of the head, and tie it to the side of device.
○ Evaluate and adjust the straps. They must be tight enough so the device does not move excessively up, down, left, or right, but not so tight as to restrict the patient's breathing.

> **note** ———————————————————————
>
> The pelvic straps must be released after the casualty is
> placed on a long backboard.

④ Place the casualty on a long backboard.

If a backboard is not available, utilize a standard litter or improvised litter made from a board or door. A hard surface is preferable to one that gives with the casualty's weight.

○ Log-roll technique
- Place the backboard next to, and parallel with, the casualty.
- Immobilize the casualty's head and neck using manual stabilization.
  - Grasp each of the patient's shoulders, one with each hand.
  - Gently position the patient's head between your forearms.
  - Maintain manual stabilization until the casualty has been placed on the backboard.
- Apply a cervical collar, if available, or improvise one.
- Brief each of the three assistants on their duties and instruct them to kneel on the same side of the casualty, with the backboard on the opposite side of the casualty.
  - First assistant: Place the near hand on the shoulder and the far hand on the waist.
  - Second assistant: Place the near hand on the hip and the far hand on the thigh.
  - Third assistant: Place the near hand on the knee and the far hand on the ankle.
- On your command, and in unison, the assistants roll the casualty slightly toward them. Turn the casualty's head slightly, keeping it in a straight line with the spine.
- Instruct the assistants to reach across the casualty with one hand, grasp the backboard at its closest edge, and slide it against the casualty. Instruct the number two assistant to reach across the board to the far edge and hold it in place to prevent board movement.
- Instruct the assistants to slowly roll the casualty back onto the board. Keep the head and spine in a straight line.
- Place the casualty's wrists together at the waist and tie them together loosely.

note

If the cervical collar or improvised collar does not fit flush with the backboard, place a roll in the hollow space between the neck and board. The roll should only be large enough to fill the gap, not to exert pressure on the neck.

o Straddle-slide technique

> **note** _____
>
> Use the straddle-slide method when limited space makes it impossible to use the log-roll technique.

- Stand at the head of the casualty with your feet wide apart.
- Apply stabilization to the casualty's head and apply a cervical collar.
- Instruct the first assistant to stand behind you (facing your back), to line up the backboard, and to gently push the backboard under the casualty at your command.
- Instruct the second assistant to straddle the casualty while facing you and gently elevate the casualty's shoulders so that the backboard can be slid under them.
- Instruct the third assistant (facing you) to carefully elevate the casualty's hips while the backboard is being slid under the casualty.
- Instruct the fourth assistant (facing you) to carefully elevate the casualty's legs and ankles while the board is being slid into place under the casualty.

▼ WARNING

> Complete all movements simultaneously, keeping the head and spine in a straight line.

> **note** _____
>
> If the cervical collar or improvised collar does not fit flush with the backboard, place a roll in the hollow space between the neck and board. The roll should only be large enough to fill the gap, not to exert pressure on the neck.

5 Secure the casualty to the long backboard.

o Secure the casualty's head and head supports to the board with straps or cravats.

▼ WARNING

> Do not release manual stabilization until the cravats or head straps are firmly in place.

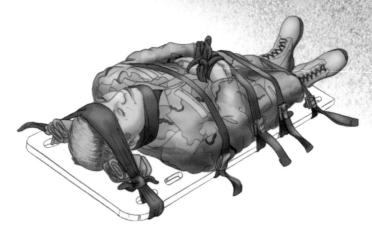

Figure 2 Using a cravat-like material across the forehead, make the supports and head one unit by tying them to the board.

- Apply head supports.
- Use two rolled towels, blankets, sandbags, or similar material.
- Place one close to each side of the head.
- Using a cravat-like material across the forehead, make the supports and head one unit by tying them to the board (**Figure 2**).
○ Secure the casualty with straps across the chest, hips, thighs, and lower legs.

note

Include the arms if the straps are long enough. If the backboard is not provided with straps and fasteners, use cravats or other long strips of cloth.

⚠ WARNING

Securely immobilize the casualty's head and neck. Fill socks with sand and place them on both sides of the head and neck to keep them from moving.

6 Record the treatment on the Field Medical Card.

7 Evacuate the casualty.

Transport: SKED Litter or Improvised Litter

Performance Steps

1 Secure the casualty to a SKED litter.

○ Remove the SKED from pack and place on ground. Unfasten the retainer strap, step on the foot end of the SKED, and unroll it completely to the opposite end.

○ Bend the SKED in half and back roll. Repeat with opposite end of litter. The SKED litter will now lay flat.

○ Place the SKED litter next to the patient. Ensure that the head end of the litter is adjacent to the head of the patient. Place cross straps under SKED.

○ Logroll the patient and slide the SKED as far under the patient as possible. Gently roll the patient down onto the SKED litter.

○ Slide the patient to the center of the SKED litter. Be sure to keep the spinal column as straight as possible.

○ Pull straps out from under SKED litter.

○ Lift the sides of the SKED and fasten the four cross straps to the buckles directly opposite the straps.

○ Lift the foot portion of the SKED and feed the foot straps through the unused grommets at the foot end of the SKED and fasten them to the buckles.

> **note** ─────────────────────────────────────
>
> The dragline is attached to the head portion of the SKED litter and is used to transport the casualty off the battlefield.

2 If a SKED litter is unavailable, gather materials to make an improvised litter.

3 Evacuate the casualty.

There are times when a patient may have to be moved and a standard litter is not available. The distance may be too great for manual carries, or the patient may have an injury that would be aggravated by manual transportation. In these situations, litters can be improvised from materials at hand. Improvised litters must be as well constructed as possible to avoid the risk of dropping or further injuring the patient. Improvised litters are emergency measures and must be replaced by standard litters at the first opportunity.

Improvised Litters

Two people can support or carry a casualty without equipment for only short distances. By using available materials to improvise equipment, the casualty can be transported greater distances by two or more rescuers.

○ Many different types of litters can be improvised, depending upon the materials available (**Figures 3 to 5**). Satisfactory litters can be made by securing poles inside such items as blankets, ponchos, shelter halves, tarpaulins, jackets, shirts, sacks, bags, and bed tickings (the fabric covers of mattresses). Poles can be improvised from strong branches, tent supports, skis, and other like items. Most flat-surface objects of suitable size can also be used as litters. Such objects include boards, doors, window shutters, benches, ladders, cots, and poles tied together. If possible, these objects should be padded.

○ If no poles can be obtained, a large item such as a blanket can be rolled from both sides toward the center. The rolls then can be used to obtain a firm grip when carrying the casualty. If a poncho is used, make sure the hood is up and under the casualty and is not dragging on the ground.

○ The important thing to remember is that an improvised litter must be well constructed to avoid the risk of dropping or further injuring the casualty.

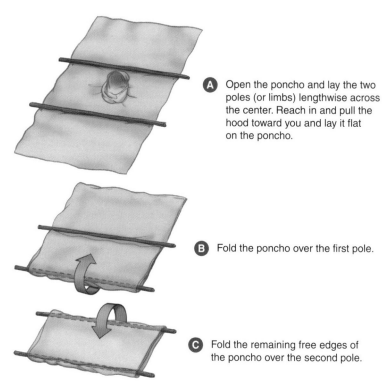

A Open the poncho and lay the two poles (or limbs) lengthwise across the center. Reach in and pull the hood toward you and lay it flat on the poncho.

B Fold the poncho over the first pole.

C Fold the remaining free edges of the poncho over the second pole.

Figure 3   Improvised litter with poncho and jacket.

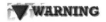 **WARNING**

Unless there is an immediate life-threatening situation (such as fire or explosion), *do not* move the casualty with a suspected back or neck injury. Seek medical personnel for guidance on how to transport.

○ Either two or four soldiers (head/foot) may be used to lift a litter. To lift the litter, follow this procedure:
  ■ Raise the litter at the same time as the other carriers or bearers.
  ■ Keep the casualty as level as possible.

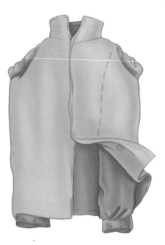

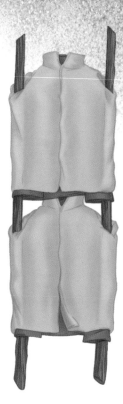

A Button two or three shirts or jackets and turn them inside out, leaving the sleeves inside.

Figure 4 Improvised litter with poles and jacket.

B Pass poles through the sleeves.

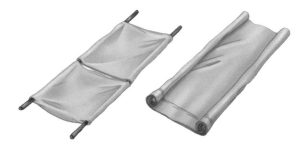

Figure 5 Improvised litters made by inserting poles through sacks or by rolling blankets.

note ————————————————————————

Use caution when transporting on an incline or hill.

Field Medical Card

Performance Steps

1 Remove the protective sheet from the carbon copy.

2 Complete the minimum required blocks.

o Block 1: Enter the casualty's name, rank, and complete Social Security number (SSN). If the casualty is a foreign military person (including prisoners of war), enter his or her military service number. Enter the casualty's military occupational specialty (MOS) or area of concentration for the specialty code. Enter the casualty's religion and sex.

o Block 3: Use the figures in the block to show the location of the injury or injuries. Check the appropriate box or boxes to describe the casualty's injury or injuries.

note ————————————————————————

Use only authorized abbreviations. Except for the following abbreviations, however, abbreviations may not be used for diagnostic terminology.

o Abr W: Abraded wound
o Cont W: Contused wound
o FC: Fracture (compound), open
o FCC: Fracture (compound), open comminuted
o FS: Fracture (simple), closed
o LW: Lacerated wound
o MW: Multiple wounds
o Pen W: Penetrating wound
o Perf W: Perforating wound
o SL: Slight
o SV: Severe

- Block 4: Check the appropriate box.
- Block 7: Check the yes or no box. Write in the dose administered and the date and time that it was administered.
- Block 9: Write in the information requested. If you need additional space, use Block 14.
- Block 11: Initial the far right side of the block.

3 Complete the other blocks as time permits. Most blocks are self-explanatory. The following specifics are noted.

- Block 2: Enter the casualty's unit of assignment and the country of whose armed forces he or she is a member. Check the armed service of the casualty, that is, A/T = Army, AF/A = Air Force, N/M = Navy, and MC/M = Marine.
- Block 5: Write in the casualty's pulse rate and the time that the pulse was measured.
- Block 6: Check the yes or no box. If a tourniquet was applied, you should write in the time and date it was applied.
- Block 8: Write in the time, date, and type of IV solution given. If you need additional space, use Block 9.
- Block 10: Check the appropriate box. Write in the date and time of disposition.
- Block 12: Write in the time and date of the casualty's arrival. Record the casualty's blood pressure, pulse, and respirations in the space provided.
- Block 13: Document the appropriate comments by the date and time of observation.
- Block 14: Document the provider's orders by date and time. Record the dose of tetanus administered and the time it was administered. Record the type and dose of antibiotic administered and the time it was administered.
- Block 15: The signature of the provider or medical officer is written in this block.
- Block 16: Check the appropriate box and enter the date and time.
- Block 17: This block will be completed by the United Ministry Team. Check the appropriate box of the service provided. The signature of the chaplain providing the service is written in this block.

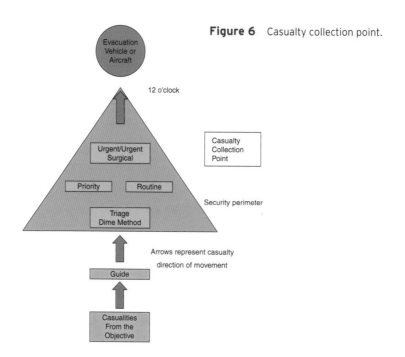

Figure 6   Casualty collection point.

Establish a Casualty Collection Point

Tactical battle plans will vary depending on the type and number of units incorporated into the plan. The plan for casualty collection points (CCPs) will vary also. The medical treatment provided on the battlefield in usually accomplished by the unit's combat medics and combat lifesavers. Point-of-wounding care is vital in saving lives on the battlefield. Establishment of a CCP is essential for the rapid treatment and evacuation of the casualty (**Figure 6**).

Performance Steps

1   Select the site.

o The location of the CCP will depend on the unit location, the tactical situation, and the number of casualties to be evacuated.

■ The location should be decided by the company or platoon medics and the unit's first sergeant.

- Battle drills and tactical standard operating procedures (TSOPs) should be established on how to get the casualty from the fighting position or vehicle to the CCP.
- The platoon CCP should be located at the platoon's rear.
- The company CCP should be located in a covered and concealed position with the company trains.
- All CCPs are identified with both day and night marking systems and contain a triage area.

② Move casualties to the CCP.

- Casualty movement from the point of wounding to the platoon CCP will be by field-expedient means, individual manual carries, litter (SKED, Talon, poleless) carries, or CASEVAC vehicle.
- Non-standard CASEVAC vehicles are positioned forward with an M996 or M997 ground ambulance designated for litter casualties at the company CCP.
- The first sergeant coordinates patient flow between the platoon CCPs and the company CCP, while the senior medic conducts triage.
- Communication of 9-line MEDEVAC requests is conducted via the company train's assets or ambulances back to the battalion aid station (BAS).
- The procedure or drill from the CCP to the BAS focuses largely on distance, routes, security, and operational procedures at the BAS.

> **note**
>
> "Operational procedures" refers to the set-up and functionality of the BAS with regard to patient flow, triage, treatment, and various other functions required for successful operation (**Figure 7**). In some cases the BAS will split into two treatment teams: the main aid station (MAS) and a forward aid station (FAS). Often the MAS and the FAS will conduct echelonment (bounding) during an offensive operation to maintain doctrinal distance during the fight. Whether evacuation is from the CCP to the MAS, FAS, or BAS, the system remains essentially the same.

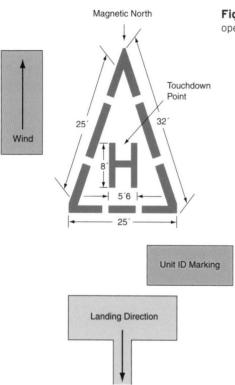

Figure 7 Semifixed base operations (day).

Magnetic North

Touchdown Point

Wind

25′ 32′

8′

5′6

25′

Unit ID Marking

Landing Direction

note

Doctrinal distance is considered to be 1 to 4 kilometers and/or one to two terrain features behind the unit supported, emphasizing mission, enemy, terrain, troops, time available, and civilian considerations (METT-TC). Failure to maintain this is a common error. Usually the distance becomes extended due to poor planning, failure to commit medical assets forward, lack of clearly defined triggers, or communications failures.

Evacuation

Categories

- Urgent/Urgent Surgical: Those casualties who will probably deteriorate without significant intervention that can be offered quickly. These casualties need evacuation within 2 hours if survival is expected.
- Priority: Those casualties who have serious injuries but who are not likely to deteriorate within the next 4 hours.
- Routine: Those casualties with injuries that are not likely to deteriorate within the next 24 hours.
- Convenience: Those casualties who have minor injuries.

Establish a Helicopter Landing Zone

Performance Steps

> **CAUTION**
>
> (1) During training, dispose of all batteries in accordance with unit SOP. (2) Comply with unit SOP and/or local regulations concerning the cutting of live vegetation, digging holes, and/or erosion prevention.

1 Select the landing site. The factors that should be considered are as follows.

- The size of the landing site
  - A helicopter requires a relatively level landing area 30 meters in diameter. This does not mean that a loaded helicopter can land and take off from an area of that size. Most helicopters cannot go straight up or down when fully loaded. Therefore, a larger landing site and better approach and departure routes are required.
  - When obstacles are in the approach or departure routes, a 10 to 1 ratio must be used to lay out the landing site. For example, during the approach and departure, if the helicopter must fly over trees that are 15 meters high, the landing site must be at least 150 meters long (10 × 15 = 150 meters).
- The ground slope of the landing site
  - When selecting the landing site, the ground slope must be no more than 15 degrees. Helicopters cannot safely land on a slope of more than 15 degrees.

- When the ground slope is under 7 degrees, the helicopter should land upslope.
- When the ground slope is 7 to 15 degrees, the helicopter must land sideslope.
○ Surface conditions
  - The ground must be firm enough that the helicopter does not bog down during loading or unloading. If firm ground cannot be found, the pilot must be told. The pilot can hover at the landing site during the loading or unloading.
  - Rotor wash on dusty, sandy, or snow-covered surfaces may cause loss of visual contact with the ground. Therefore, these areas should be avoided.
  - Loose debris that can be kicked up by the rotor wash must be removed from the landing site. Loose debris can cause damage to the helicopter blades or engines.
○ Obstacles
  - Landing sites should be free of tall trees, telephone lines, power lines or poles, and similar obstructions on the approach or departure ends of the landing site.
  - Obstructions that cannot be removed (such as large rocks, stumps, or holes) must be marked clearly within the landing site.

2 Establish security for the landing site. Landing sites should offer some security from enemy observation and direct fire. Good landing sites will allow the helicopter to land and depart without exposing it to unneeded risks. Security is normally established around the entire landing site.

3 Mark the landing site and touchdown point.

○ When and how the landing site should be marked is based on the mission, capabilities, and situation of the unit concerned. Normally, the only marks or signals required are smoke (colored) and a signalman. VS-17 marker panels may be used to mark the landing site, but *must not* be used any closer than 50 feet to the touchdown point. In addition to identifying the landing site, smoke gives the pilot information on the wind direction and speed.
○ At night, the landing site and touchdown point are marked by an inverted "Y" composed of four lights. Strobe lights, flashlights, or vehicle lights may also be used to mark the landing site. The marking system used should be fully explained to the pilot when contact is made.

Rescue and Transportation Procedures

Overview

A basic principle of first aid is to treat casualties before moving them. However, adverse situations or conditions may jeopardize the lives of both the rescuer and the casualty if this is done. It may first be necessary to rescue the casualties before first aid can be effectively or safely given. The life and/or the well-being of the casualties will depend as much upon the manner in which they are rescued and transported as upon the treatment they receive. Rescue actions must be done quickly and safely. Careless or rough handling of casualties during rescue operations can aggravate their injuries and possibly cause death.

Principles of Rescue Operations

- When faced with the necessity of rescuing a casualty who is threatened by hostile action, fire, water, or any other immediate hazard, *do not* take action without first determining the extent of the hazard and your ability to handle the situation. *Do not* become a casualty.
- The rescuer must evaluate the situation and analyze the factors involved. This evaluation involves three major steps:
  - Identify the task.
  - Evaluate the circumstances of the rescue.
  - Plan the action.

Task (Rescue) Identification

First determine if a rescue attempt is actually needed. It is a waste of time, equipment, and personnel to rescue someone not in need of rescuing. It is also a waste to look for someone who is not lost or needlessly risk the lives of the rescuers. In planning a rescue, attempt to obtain the answers to the following questions:

- Who, what, where, when, why, and how did the situation happen?
- How many casualties are involved and what is the nature of their injuries?
- What is the tactical situation?
- What are the terrain features and the location of the casualties?
- Will there be adequate assistance available to aid in the rescue and/or evacuation?
- Can treatment be provided at the scene or will the casualties require movement to a safer location?

○ What equipment will be required for the rescue operation?

○ Will decontamination procedures and equipment be required for casualties, rescue personnel, and rescue equipment?

Circumstances of the Rescue

○ After identifying the job (task) required, you must relate it to the circumstances under which you must work. Do you need additional people, security, or medical or special rescue equipment? Are there circumstances, such as mountain rescues or aircraft accidents, that may require specialized skills? What is the weather like? Is the terrain hazardous? How much time is available?

○ The time element will sometimes cause a rescuer to compromise planning stages and/or the treatment that can be given. A realistic estimate of time available must be made as quickly as possible to determine the action time remaining. The key elements are the casualty's condition and the environment.

○ Mass casualties are to be expected on the modern battlefield. All problems or complexities of rescue are now multiplied by the number of casualties encountered. In this case, time becomes the critical element.

Plan of Action

○ The casualty's ability to endure is of primary importance in estimating the time available. Age and physical condition will differ from casualty to casualty. Therefore, to determine the time available, you will have to consider the following factors:
  ■ Endurance time of the casualty
  ■ Type of situation
  ■ Personnel and/or equipment availability
  ■ Weather
  ■ Terrain

○ In respect to terrain, you must consider altitude and visibility. In some cases, the casualty may be of assistance because of knowing more about the particular terrain or situation than you do. The maximum use of secure and reliable trails or roads is essential.

○ When taking weather into account, ensure that blankets and/or rain gear are available. Even a mild rain can complicate a normally simple rescue. In high altitudes and/or extreme cold and gusting winds, the time available is critically shortened.

○ High altitudes and gusting winds minimize the ability of fixed-wing or rotary-wing aircraft to assist in operations. Rotary-wing aircraft may be available to remove casualties from cliffs or inaccessible sites.

These same aircraft can also transport the casualties to a medical treatment facility in a comparatively short time. Aircraft, though vital elements of search, rescue, or evacuation, cannot be used in all situations. For this reason, do not rely entirely on their presence. Reliance on aircraft or specialized equipment is a poor substitute for careful planning.

Mass Casualties

In situations where there are multiple casualties, an orderly rescue may involve some additional planning. To facilitate a mass casualty rescue or evacuation, recognize separate stages.

- First stage: Remove those personnel who are not trapped among debris or who can be evacuated easily.
- Second stage: Remove those personnel who may be trapped by debris but require only the equipment on hand and a minimum amount of time.
- Third stage: Remove the remaining personnel who are trapped in extremely difficult or time-consuming situations, such as under large amounts of debris or behind walls.
- Fourth stage: Remove the dead.

Proper Handling of Casualties

- You may have saved the casualty's life through the application of appropriate first aid measures. However, the casualty's life can be lost through rough handling or careless transportation procedures. Before you attempt to move the casualty:
  - Evaluate the type and extent of injury.
  - Ensure that dressings over wounds are adequately reinforced.
  - Ensure that fractured bones are properly immobilized and supported to prevent them from cutting through muscle, blood vessels, and skin.
- Based upon your evaluation of the type and extent of the casualty's injury and your knowledge of the various manual carries, you must select the best possible method of manual transportation. If the casualties are conscious, tell them how they are to be transported. This will help allay their fear of movement and gain their cooperation and confidence.
- Buddy-aid for chemical agent casualties includes those actions required to prevent an incapacitated casualty from receiving additional injury from the effects of chemical hazards. If casualties are

physically unable to decontaminate themselves or administer the proper chemical agent antidote, the casualties' buddies must assist them and assume responsibility for their care. Buddy-aid includes the following:

- Administering the proper chemical agent antidote
- Decontaminating the incapacitated casualty's exposed skin
- Ensuring that his or her protective ensemble remains correctly emplaced
- Maintaining respiration
- Controlling bleeding
- Providing other standard first aid measures
- Transporting the casualty out of the contaminated area

Transportation of Casualties

○ Transportation of the sick and wounded is the responsibility of medical personnel who have been provided special training and equipment. Therefore, unless a good reason for you to transport a casualty arises, wait for some means of medical evacuation to be provided. When the situation is urgent and you are unable to obtain medical assistance or know that no medical evacuation facilities are available, you will have to transport the casualty. For this reason, you must know how to transport a casualty without increasing the seriousness of his or her condition.

○ Transporting a casualty by litter (FM 8-35) is safer and more comfortable for a casualty than transporting by manual means; it is also easier for you. Manual transportation, however, may be the only feasible method because of the terrain or the combat situation, or it may be necessary to save a life. In these situations, the casualty should be transferred to a litter as soon as one can be made available or improvised.

Combat Convoy Operations

Operation Iraqi Freedom (OIF)/Operation Enduring Freedom (OEF) Theater Threats

○ General theater threats
- Vehicle-borne improvised explosive devices (VBIEDs)
- Suicide bombers
- Rocket-propelled grenades (RPGs)
- Sniper fire

- Direct-fire ambushes
- Grenade attacks
- Mortar attacks
- Hostile crowds
- Terrorist/hostile surveillance
- Potential specific threats
  - Locations and vehicles
    - Entrances to alleys
    - Rooftops and balconies (near and far)
    - Overpasses
    - Vans with sliding doors
    - Motorcycles
    - Ambulances
  - Personnel
    - Large crowds
    - Any person who appears not to fit in with the crowd or avoids eye contact
- Characteristics for defending against threats
  - Aggressiveness
    - Use aggressive, not "home town," driving skills.
    - "Porcupine" muzzles in an outward posture (everyone except the driver faces outward).
    - Maintain a predatory presence; "Go ahead, make my day" attitude.
    - Demonstrate a positive readiness and willingness to engage threats.
    - Consider the potential use of vehicles as weapons.
    - Dominate your environment.
  - Situational awareness (SA)
    - Maintain 360-degree security.
    - Use advance parties/reconnaissance.
    - Know your route(s).
    - Gather and use collective mission knowledge.
    - Internal communication should be well rehearsed.
    - Communicate to a higher level (Blue Force Tracker [BFT]).
    - Scan in three dimensions (depth, width, elevation).
    - Watch people, their hands, and their behavior.
  - Unpredictability
    - Adapt to an already elusive and adaptive enemy.
    - Vary routes, departure times, vehicle intervals, and vehicle speeds.
    - Think like the enemy: "How would I attack me?"

- Convoys should not be easily timed, observed, or approached.
- Do not appear lost.
■ Agility
- Drive as fast as appropriate.
- Maneuver through or around motorists, pedestrians, and so forth.
- Compress or expand vehicle intervals.
- Be prepared to rapidly change course of action with well-rehearsed SOPs and battle drills.

Improvised Explosive Devices

Improvised explosive devices (IEDs) are the greatest threats to convoys. Extremist groups continue to use IEDs to attack coalition forces in an attempt to discredit security efforts.

Types of IED Attacks

Figures 8 and 9 illustrate types of IED attacks.

> **note**
>
> IEDs can be hidden in trash or debris as well as in vehicles.

How to Protect Yourself

- Stay alert; make yourself a "hard target."
- Be prepared for an IED attack followed by an ambush.
- In the rush to aid comrades, be cautious. Do not overlook the potential for a second IED attack.
- Be and appear vigilant; personnel who look ready to fight back make bad targets.

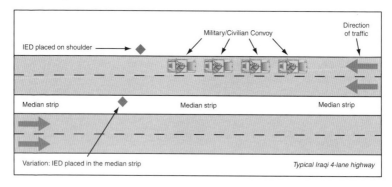

Figure 8 Typical improvised explosive device configurations.

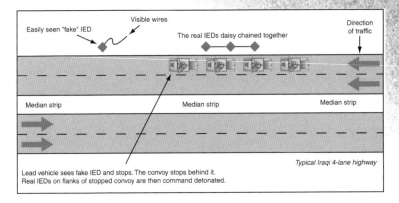

Figure 9 Multiple improvised explosive device attack.

- Maintain maximum safe speeds.
- Maintain vehicle dispersion.
- Be extra cautious at choke points: Iraqi vehicle breakdowns, bridges, one-way roads, traffic jams, and sharp turns.
- If something causes the convoy to stop, watch the flanks for IEDs; dismount with weapons at the ready.
- Vests and helmets save lives: Wear them!
- Ballistic eye protection saves eyesight.
- Rehearse actions for contact with an IED.
- Get out of the "kill zone" fast.
- Do not approach the IED; IEDs are often command-detonated.
- Brief all convoy personnel on the latest IED threat, what types of IEDs are being used, and where they have previously been placed on your route.

Field Sanitation

The Medical Threat

The impact of casualties caused by disease and nonbattle injuries (DNBI) on military campaigns has been a prominent and continuous feature of military operations. From the beginning of recorded history up to the present time, armies have had immense problems with heat, cold, and communicable diseases. In all U.S. conflicts, three times as many soldiers have been lost to DNBI as to enemy action. The ultimate objective of a military force—success in battle—demands that troops be maintained in a constant state of good health.

The three major components of the medical threat to field forces are environmental factors, zoonotic diseases and animal bites, and diseases endemic to the area of operations.

- Environmental factors: These include humidity, significant elevations above sea level, and, of course, heat and cold. Of these, heat and cold are the most significant.
  - Heat is the most lethal component of all. Those of us born and raised in temperate climates have a hard time relating to heat and its awesome impact. During the 1967 Arab-Israeli conflict, the Israelis enveloped the Egyptians, severing their lines of support. The Egyptians suffered 20,000 deaths due to heat, whereas the Israelis had no deaths and only 128 cases of heat injury. The Israelis demonstrated that health hazards, such as heat, could be as effective as tactical weapons in securing success on the battlefield.

    Commanders can minimize the effects of heat by ensuring that soldiers drink adequate amounts of water. Remember that thirst is a poor indicator of a body's need for water. Commanders should also ensure that soldiers consume three meals a day to replace lost electrolytes and, when the tactical situation permits, follow correct work/rest cycles.
  - Cold weather can also be very incapacitating on the battlefield. In World War II, during the winter of 1944-45 in the European theater, over 54,000 U.S. soldiers were admitted to hospitals with cold injuries. Over 90,000 U.S. soldiers were admitted with cold injuries throughout the war.

    Commanders can reduce the rate of cold injuries by incorporating weather data into operations planning; enforcing the proper wearing of the uniform; ensuring that soldiers frequently change damp socks; and, when the tactical situation permits, providing warming areas.
- Zoonotic diseases and animal bites
  - Many species of arthropods transmit diseases that can seriously affect military operations. Napoleon's Grand Armee numbered over 500,000 when it crossed the Russian border in June of 1812. Although he reached Moscow in the winter as the Russians pulled back, disease and cold injury decimated Napoleon's troops as his army retreated to Paris, returning with fewer than 20,000 men. There were approximately 70,000 combat losses and 400,000

DNBI losses. It is estimated that over 100,000 of Napoleon's soldiers were lost to louse-borne typhus.

Commanders must ensure that soldiers use the Department of Defense (DOD) Insect Repellent System (33% DEET on skin, permethrin on uniforms, and proper wear of the uniform); use bed nets when appropriate; and consume prescribed prophylactic medications when necessary.

○ Diseases endemic to the area of operations
  ■ Of these endemic diseases, diarrheal disease can be contracted from contaminated water or food; in either case, it can have a catastrophic impact on the fighting force. Rommel's situation in North Africa is a superb example. Not one of Rommel's original highly successful generals was available to help him when he needed them most—that is, at El Alamein; they had all, over time, been medically evacuated for illness. Rommel himself was not present when the battle began; he was in Germany recovering from hepatitis. His chief of staff and his intelligence officer were evacuated just before the battle, and his operations officer was evacuated during the battle—all three for amebic dysentery. In Operation Bright Star in 1980, the U.S. commander rewarded his troops for a job well done by allowing them to go into town the evening prior to redeployment. Thirty percent of his command contracted shigellosis and were simultaneously vomiting and defecating in the aircraft on the flight back to the states. These examples are just as relevant today as in the past.

Commanders must ensure that soldiers only consume food and water from approved sources, that waste disposal and hand washing devices are constructed, and that unit dining facilities are operated under sanitary conditions.

Soldier Health

The direct relationship between soldier health and success in battle must be emphasized throughout the chain of command. Commanders must gain a new awareness of the importance of preventive medicine (PVNTMED). With sound preventive medicine measures (PMM), an army can maintain its fighting strength and exploit that strength when the enemy expects weakness.

In the field, soldiers have increased vulnerability to DNBI because of the following:

○ The harshness of the environment and the tactical situation. The operational environment may be infested with mosquitoes, sand flies, or other disease-carrying pests; it may be a hot, dusty desert or a cold, windy plain. Soldiers and their leaders must be prepared to live and fight in such places.

○ The disruption of the body's natural defenses. The human body has an excellent capacity to protect itself against disease and climatic injury; however, the efficiency of these mechanisms is dependent upon an individual's overall well-being. Deploying soldiers halfway around the world disrupts their personal biological rhythms. The addition of heat or cold, meals served at irregular hours, and sleep deprivation soon results in soldiers who are more susceptible to illness and combat stress. Additionally, because soldiers have not been exposed to the diseases present in many deployment areas, they are more susceptible to becoming seriously ill from these diseases than the native population. Vector-borne disease may present a hidden threat to deploying units. Immunologically naïve soldiers may be at more risk from vector-borne disease than the local populace due to the local populace's relatively higher immunity to them. There may be the mistaken impression that the disease threat is low when it is high for the deployed units; therefore, PMM are essential on all deployments.

○ Breakdowns in basic sanitation. Potable water and proper waste disposal are examples of things taken for granted in garrison. Using the latrine or changing your socks becomes a challenge when one is living in a muddy foxhole.

○ Consumption of unauthorized rations, including locally procured and scavenged food.

The Individual in a Field Environment

Ordinarily, the U.S. soldier has a high standard of personal hygiene when in an environment with convenient facilities. In the field, however, where proper sanitation requires coping with the elements of nature, a problem arises: The soldier is suddenly faced with inconveniences.

In garrison, soldiers readily conduct daily personal hygiene. Routine acts of personal hygiene are performed in a conveniently located latrine that is warm and has hot and cold water. However, upon arising in the field, a soldier may feel too cold to change into clean underwear. Even in the summer, a cold-water shower is uncomfortable. Usually, the toilet in the field is not as pleasant as the one in garrison. An ordinarily well-groomed individual may become dirty and unkempt. Filth and disease go hand in hand. Dirty, sweaty socks may cause feet to be more susceptible to disease. Dirty clothing worn for prolonged periods of time and unwashed hair are open invitations to lice. In addition to keeping uniforms clean, treating them with clothing repellent will prevent body louse infestations.

The problems entailed in reducing DNBI, therefore, pertain not only to the existing elements of nature but also to the reactions of soldiers brought into the environment. Inadequate individual PMM in the field is one of the most difficult problems to overcome because it requires a sense of responsibility on the part of each individual to try to maintain his or her health regardless of the difficulties encountered.

Preventive Medicine Measures

Arthropod and Rodent Control

○ Ensure that proper waste disposal is practiced. It is essential for arthropod and rodent control and is in compliance with applicable environmental laws.

○ Explain to soldiers the ways in which arthropods may affect their health, and instruct them to use PMM.

○ Apply pesticides as required for arthropod control. Be sure to follow product label instructions exactly.

○ Inspect to ensure the elimination of food and shelter for rodents.

○ Use traps and authorized rodenticides as required in the control of rodents.

○ Report deficiencies to the field service team (FST) or the unit commander.

Personal Hygiene

○ The FST can promote the personal hygiene of soldiers by arranging for facilities such as hand-washing and showering devices, hot water for shaving, and a heated place to dress. Hand-washing devices are provided outside latrine enclosures and in the food service area. They may also be set up at other points in the bivouac area. They are constructed so that they operate easily. They must be kept filled with water at all times. All hand-washing and showering devices must have a soakage pit underneath them to prevent water from collecting and forming pools.

○ Ensure that soldiers understand and receive guidance as needed concerning the hazards involved when personal hygiene is neglected. Inspect soldiers to ensure adequate personal hygiene, including body, hair, and teeth; airing sleeping bags; wearing clean clothes (including socks); and disposing of refuse. Enforcement of sanitary control measures pertaining to all camp facilities encourages soldiers to have more pride in their personal hygiene.

Water

○ General importance
- Water is essential to the army in the field. Safe water ranks in importance with ammunition and food as a unit of supply in combat and often has an important bearing on the success or failure of a mission.
- When in the field, soldiers must be supplied with sufficient potable water to drink and for personal hygiene (such as shaving, brushing teeth, helmet baths, and comfort cleaning). The water for these purposes must be safe for human consumption and should be reasonably free of objectionable tastes, odors, turbidity, and color. For showering, disinfected nonpotable fresh water is to be used. However, only potable water will be used for showering, bathing, or bodily contact in the following locations:
  - Where diseases such as schistosomiasis and leptospirosis are endemic and prevalent
  - Where chemical agents may be present
○ Water as a vehicle in disease transmission
- Waterborne disease organisms are a primary source of illness to soldiers. Common waterborne diseases of man include hepatitis, typhoid, and paratyphoid fever, bacillary and amebic dysentery, cholera, common diarrhea, leptospirosis, and schistosomiasis (snail fever).
- No direct method has been developed for detecting the minimum infectious quantities of these organisms in water; therefore, it is necessary to resort to an indicator test to determine the bacteriologic acceptability of water. The water is tested for the presence of coliform bacteria.
- Coliform bacteria are found in great numbers in the excreta (feces) of humans and warm-blooded animals, and in the soil. Also, many of the diseases mentioned earlier are spread through feces.
- Although the presence of coliform bacteria in water may not prove fecal contamination, it is an indication that pathogenic (disease-carrying) organisms may be present. The indicator test is the best sign that contamination exists; therefore, we must assume that pathogens are present.
- Many military units in the field do not have the capability for determining the presence of coliform bacteria in water; hence, all water must be thoroughly treated and disinfected before use.

- Quantity of water required for soldiers: The quantity of water required for soldiers varies with the season of the year, the geographic area, and the tactical situation.
  - In a cold climate, only 2 gallons of water per soldier per day may be required for drinking purposes even though soldiers are engaged in physical activity.
  - In a hot climate, 3 or 4 gallons of water per soldier per day may be required when soldiers are engaged in only sedentary duty.
  - Additional amounts of water are required for personal hygiene and cooking. A guide for meeting the water requirements in an arid zone is to plan for 3 to 6 gallons per individual per day unless improvised showering facilities are made available. In this case, the requirement should be increased to 15 gallons or more.

> **note**
>
> For additional information on water requirements, see FM 10-52.

Waste Disposal

The proper disposal of all wastes is essential in preventing the spread of diseases. Liquid and solid wastes produced under field conditions may amount to 100 pounds per person per day, especially when shower facilities are available. A camp or bivouac area without proper waste disposal methods soon becomes an ideal breeding ground for flies, rats, and other vermin and may result in diseases such as dysentery (amebic and bacillary), typhoid, paratyphoid, and cholera among soldiers.

- Responsibilities for waste disposal
  - The unit commander is responsible for proper waste disposal in his or her unit area. Commanders should check with the Logistics Officer (S4) or the supporting PVNTMED officer for assistance with the removal of hazardous waste.
  - The PVNTMED personnel are responsible for inspecting waste facilities and methods of operation. These personnel recommend changes that aid in protecting the health and welfare of soldiers.
- Types of waste requiring disposal
  - Human waste (feces and urine)
  - Animal waste
  - Garbage

- Kitchen and bath liquid waste
- Rubbish
- Hazardous waste

o Waste disposal methods: The methods selected for use will depend upon the location of the unit and the military situation. Generally, wastes are buried if the environment (especially soil conditions) and local regulations permit.

o Field facilities for human waste disposal
   - Human waste disposal becomes a problem for both the individual and the unit in the field. Local, state, federal, and host-nation regulations or laws may prohibit burning or burial of waste.
   - Chemical latrines are the preferred human waste disposal devices for use during field exercises or missions. If possible, urinals should be provided in these facilities to prevent soiling the toilet seats. The number of latrines is based on a calculation of one commode or urinal per 25 male soldiers and one commode per 17 female soldiers.
   - When chemical latrines are not available, individuals and units must use improvised devices. During short halts when troops are on a march, each soldier uses a brief relief bag or "cat-hole" latrine. The cat-hole latrine is dug approximately 1 foot deep and is completely covered and packed down after use. In temporary bivouac areas (1 to 3 days), the straddle trench latrine is used unless more permanent facilities are provided for the unit. When setting up a temporary camp, a deep-pit latrine and urine soakage pits are usually constructed.
   - Alternate devices that may be used to dispose of human waste in the field are the burn-out, mound, bored-hole, or pail latrines (see FM 21-10). The burn-out latrine is the preferred method for improvised devices.

Arthropods and Diseases

Arthropods (insects, ticks, mites, spiders, scorpions, and the like) make up over 75% of all animal species. Fewer than 1% of the 750,000 species of arthropods are potentially dangerous to humans. The impact of all arthropods is significant because of their high numbers and the negative results of their infestation of stored products and wooden structures. Still, many species are beneficial as pollinators, predators of other pests, scavengers of waste, and manufacturers of food and are a part of the natural balance of nature. However, the economic damage and medical disorders caused by a few arthropods make some pest management practices necessary to control the problem pests.

Historically, arthropod-borne diseases have caused more casualties than combat injuries. Arthropod-borne diseases alone were responsible for the loss of 15,576,000 man-days among the U.S. Armed Forces during World War II. Today, harmful arthropods represent one of the greatest environmental hazards to soldiers in the field. Protection of the soldier from arthropods and arthropod-borne diseases is essential to mission accomplishment. See the PVNTMED team for effective arthropod control measures.

○ The chain of infection for arthropod-borne diseases involves a pathogenic organism in an infected person or animal (the reservoir), an arthropod to transmit the disease (the vector), and a susceptible person (the host).

○ The efficiency of the vector in transmitting disease from a reservoir to a host is related to many factors. Some of the factors are species related, such as vector reproductive capacity, physiology, morphology, and genetics. Other factors that affect the vector's ability to transmit disease are physical and related to environmental conditions, such as temperature, moisture, rainfall, pH, weather, geographic and topographic location, photoperiod, and wind.

○ Soldiers in a field environment must break the chain of infection for arthropod-borne disease or arthropod injury by limiting arthropod pest exposures.

Direct Arthropod Effects on Human Health

In addition to disease transmission, arthropods can cause direct injuries to people. Bites, stings, and allergic reactions are three major categories of injuries caused by arthropods. Arthropods also affect humans by annoying and disturbing them. The sound of a single mosquito buzzing around your head while you are trying to sleep is annoying. Standing guard with gnats buzzing around your face can be disturbing. Finding cockroaches or other insects or parts of insects in your food is disturbing. The problems of arthropod injury and the exaggerated fear of arthropods can even result in psychiatric problems.

Arthropod-borne Diseases

The diseases transmitted to man by arthropods are some of the most serious known to man. Uncontrolled, these illnesses can cripple or destroy military forces. The effect of these diseases on man can range from a very mild illness to a severe illness or death. For examples of arthropod-borne diseases and their vectors, see **Table 3**. House flies

Table 3	Arthropod-borne Diseases and Their Vectors
Disease	**Vector**
Malaria	Mosquito
Chagas' disease	Kissing bug (reduvid)
Leishmaniasis	Sand fly (phlebotomine)
Yellow fever	Mosquito
Dengue fever	Mosquito
Encephalitis	Mosquito
Sandfly fever or phlebotomus fever	Sand fly (phlebotomine)
Typhus fever (epidemic)	Body louse
Typhus fever (murine)	Flea
Scrub typhus	Larval mite
Bubonic plague	Flea
Dysentery	Filth flies (particularly the house fly)
Typhoid fever	Flies and cockroaches (by food contamination)
Spotted fever	Tick
Filariasis (elephantiasis)	Mosquito
Onchocerciasis	Black fly

and other flying insects that are attracted to human wastes or other organic material can spread disease organisms to food and water. The disease organisms or parasites of humans are carried from diseased humans or animals (reservoirs) by arthropods (vectors) to humans or animals (hosts). By employing individual PMM, soldiers can stop arthropod-borne diseases from being a factor in their lives and in their unit's mission accomplishment.

Arthropod Control

Bivouac sites are selected according to well-defined guidelines. The ideal location for a bivouac site is on high, well-drained ground at least 1 mile from breeding sites of flies and mosquitoes and 1 mile from native habitations. It is not always possible to bivouac in the ideal location. A unit commander may be faced with unusual arthropod control problems in the vicinity of the campsite. An effective program for arthropod-borne disease prevention should consist primarily of sanitation measures, but may include the use of individual PMM, such as bed nets, as well as the application of pesticides. Essential to the operation of an effective control program is an understanding of the life cycles of medically important arthropods and knowledge of where they can be found in nature. For more information, refer to FM 4-25.12 (FM 21-10-1), or see the unit preventive medicine team.

Preventive Medicine Measures for Arthropods

Individual PMM are those measures that must be used by each soldier. Often they are the only preventive measures available for soldiers in the field. These PMM can be accomplished by the soldier at work and at rest.

- The DOD Insect Repellent System: The best strategy for defense against insects and other disease-bearing arthropods is use of the DOD Insect Repellent System. This system includes the application of extended-duration 33% DEET repellent to exposed skin, the application of permethrin to the field uniform, and a properly worn uniform. When used correctly, the DOD Insect Repellent System can provide nearly complete protection from arthropod-borne disease.
- It is important to note that not all arthropod species are equally repelled by a particular repellent, so a soldier should not discontinue using repellents if some bites are received, because other species that are present are still likely to be repelled. Further, some insect species bite primarily during the day, whereas others do so only at night. This is true even within a pest group like mosquitoes; therefore, a lack of bites during the day does not mean that protective measures will not be needed at night.

Food

General

- Factors that create a high risk for foodborne diseases include poor food inspection and sanitation, poor personal hygiene habits, inadequate refrigeration, and lack of eradication programs for foodborne diseases such as hepatitis A and brucellosis.
- Food transportation, storage, preparation, and service have direct bearing on the success or failure of a mission. Dining facility sanitation is a chronic operational problem. The prospect of disease outbreaks, particularly dysentery and food poisoning, is always present and must be recognized as a constant threat to unit health.
- Potentially hazardous foods (PHFs) are any food that contains milk, milk products, eggs, meat, poultry, fish, shellfish, or other ingredients in a form capable of supporting the rapid growth of infectious or toxic microorganisms. PHFs are typically high in protein and have a water content greater than 85% and a pH greater than 4.5.
- Factors that most often cause foodborne disease outbreaks:
  - Failure to keep PHFs cold (below 40°F [4.4°C] internal temperature)
  - Failure to keep PHFs hot (above 145°F [62.8°C] internal temperature)
  - Preparing foods a day or more before serving
  - Allowing sick employees who practice poor personal hygiene to handle food

- Food contamination can be classified into three categories:
  - Biological: Contamination by pathogenic microorganisms (protozoa, bacteria, fungus, virus) or unacceptable levels of spoilage. This category is the major threat to personnel.
  - Chemical: Contamination with chemical warfare agents, industrial chemicals, and/or other adulterating chemicals (zinc, copper, cadmium, pesticides, etc.).
  - Physical: Contamination by arthropods, debris, radioactive particles, etc.
- Bacteria that multiply at temperatures between 60°F (15.5°C) and 125°F (52°C) cause most foodborne illness. Maintain the internal temperature of cooked foods that will be served hot at 145°F (63°C) or above. Maintain the internal temperatures of foods that will be served cold at 40°F (4.4°C) or below to control any bacteria that may be present in the food.
- The high food temperatures (160°F to 212°F [71°C to 100°C]) reached in boiling, baking, frying, and roasting will kill most bacteria that can cause foodborne illness. Prompt refrigeration to 40°F (4.4°C) or below in containers less than 2 inches deep inhibits growth of most (but not all) of these bacteria. Freezing at 0°F (-18°C) or below essentially stops bacteria growth but will not kill bacteria that are already present.
- Thorough reheating to an internal temperature of 165°F (74°C) or above will kill bacteria that may have grown during storage. However, foods that have been improperly stored or otherwise mishandled cannot be made safe by reheating.
- Ensure that everything that touches food during preparation and serving is clean to avoid introducing illness-causing bacteria.

Procurement of Food

- Order of preference for food acquisition:
  - U.S. military rations brought with unit or previously cached
  - Local food procured from sources approved by supporting Veterinary and Environmental Science Officers
  - Local food procured from unapproved sources
- Special Operations Forces will probably have to procure food from unapproved sources during real-world contingencies, presenting a serious medical threat to the team and the mission. Use the following guidelines:
  - Avoid local street vendors. Their personal hygiene habits tend to be poor, which results in contaminated food (e.g., through fecal-oral contamination).

- Consider all ice contaminated. It is often made from nonpotable water, and freezing will not kill disease-causing organisms. Anything with ice in it or on it should be considered contaminated (e.g., alcohol in a drink does not make the ice in it safe).
- Semi-perishable rations (canned and dried products) are relatively safe and should be chosen over fresh food. Protect canned and dried foods from extreme heating and freezing. Do not use swollen or leaking cans. Do not procure moldy grain or grain contaminated with insect larvae.
- Be aware that raw fruit and vegetables may be grown in areas where "nightsoil" (human fecal matter) is used as fertilizer or where gastrointestinal or parasitic diseases are prevalent. Wash raw fresh fruits and vegetables in potable water and disinfect with one of the following methods.
  - Dip in boiling water for 15 seconds: Place small amounts of produce in net bags, completely submerge items for 15 seconds, and then remove and allow cooling. This method is not recommended for leafy vegetables.
  - Disinfect with chlorine: Immerse for at least 15 minutes in a 100 parts per million (ppm) solution of chlorine or for 30 minutes in a 50 ppm solution (see **Table 4**). Rinse the produce thoroughly with potable water before cooking or eating. Break apart "head" produce such as lettuce, cabbage, or celery before disinfection.
- Always cook eggs to prevent salmonellosis. Blood and meat spots are acceptable, but cracked and rotten eggs are not acceptable and should be discarded.
- Boil unpasteurized dairy products for at least 15 seconds to prevent tuberculosis, brucellosis, Q fever, and so forth. Avoid cheese, butter, and ice cream made from unpasteurized milk, which can carry these diseases.

Table 4	Bleach Solutions
Chlorox	
4.84 oz in 32 gallons = 50 ppm	
9.68 oz in 32 gallons = 100 ppm	
1 tablespoon per gallon = 200 ppm	
70% Calcium hypochlorite	
0.32 oz in 32 gallons = 50 ppm	
0.64 oz in 32 gallons = 100 ppm	

- Cook all seafood to prevent hepatitis, tapeworms, flukes, cholera, and so forth.
  - Avoid shellfish-cooking does not degrade some toxins (e.g., red tide).
  - Certain saltwater fish have heat-stable toxins that are not destroyed during cooking. Do not eat any species that the native population does not eat.
  - Avoid large predatory reef fish, such as barracuda, grouper, snapper, jack, mackerel, and triggerfish, which may accumulate toxins (e.g., ciguatera).
  - Be aware of geographic areas where toxins may occur in seafood.
- Eat carcass or muscle meat rather than visceral meat (liver, heart, kidney, etc.). Muscle flesh is less likely to be contaminated. Fresh meat from healthy animals is safe if cooked thoroughly.
  - Perform an antemortem examination (before slaughtering), use correct field slaughter methods, and perform a postmortem examination (after slaughtering).
  - The color of meat should be red to slightly red-brown. Do not consume green or brown beef if possible. Avoid meat with off odors, such as sour or sweet, fruity smells.
  - Cook meat until it is *well done:* Do not eat rare, medium, or bloody meat. Sausages and meat products should be well cooked.

Food Storage and Preservation

- Protect canned and dried foods from extreme heat and freezing.
- Store and preserve perishables such as meat, poultry, and fish by refrigerating at or below 40ºF (4.4ºC). Because refrigeration or potable ice is often not available, slaughter what you need, cook it thoroughly, and then consume it immediately. Meat can be preserved by methods other than refrigeration (e.g., by smoking, curing, making jerky or pemmican, salting, or pickling) if time and resources are available.
- Semi-perishable foods such as potatoes and onions should be stored in a dry place off the ground, allowing air to circulate around them to retard decay and spoilage.
- Store staple products (flour, sugar, etc.) in metal cans with tight-fitting lids.
- Do not store acidic foods or beverages such as tomatoes or citric juices in galvanized cans. This will prevent zinc poisoning.

Preparing and Serving Food

- Use pesticides according to the directions on the container. Limit residual sprays to crack and crevice treatment only. Protect all foods and food contact surfaces when applying pesticides.

- Coordinate food preparation and consumption to eliminate unnecessary lapses of time.
- Leftover food presents a problem. Plan meals to reduce the amount of leftovers. Discard items held at unsafe temperatures (45ºF to 140ºF [7.2ºC to 60ºC]) for 3 or more hours. Never save potentially hazardous foods such as creamed beef, casseroles, or gravies.
- Meat may contain disease-producing agents that cannot be detected by inspection. Follow cooking procedures strictly to ensure that heat penetrates to the center of the meat and that all the meat is cooked to at least 165ºF (74ºC). This applies to poultry, pork, beef, and any stuffing or other foods containing these meats.

Cleaning and Disinfecting Utensils

- Cooking utensils and mess kits should be cleaned, disinfected, and properly stored after each use. They must be scraped free of food particles, washed in hot (120ºF to 130ºF [49ºC to 54ºC]) soapy water, rinsed in boiling water, sanitized for at least 10 seconds in another container of boiling water, and allowed to air dry. They must be stored in clean, covered containers that are protected from dust and vermin.
- When it is impossible to heat the water, utensils must be washed in soapy water, rinsed in two cans of clear water, and then immersed in a fourth container of chlorine sanitizing solution for at least 30 seconds. Chemical sanitizing solutions are prepared as followed (methods are listed in the order of preference).
  - Use Disinfectant, Food Service (NSN: 6840-01-035-5432) as specified on the label.
  - Use 1 level mess kit spoonful of calcium hypochlorite for every 10 gallons of water (250 ppm solution).
  - Use 1 canteen cup of 5% liquid bleach in 32 gallons of water (250 ppm solution).
- If mess kits become soiled or contaminated between meals, they should be rewashed prior to use as described previously. A prewash of boiling water should be available for use prior to all meals

Water

Fill your canteen with treated water at every chance. When treated water is not available, you must disinfect the water in your canteen using one of the following methods.

- Preferred method: Iodine tablets
  - Fill your canteen with the cleanest water available.
  - Put two iodine tablets in the canteen of water. Double these amounts in the 2-quart canteen.

- Place cap on canteen. Shake canteen to dissolve tablets. Wait 5 minutes. Loosen the cap and tip the canteen over to allow leakage around the canteen threads. Tighten the cap and wait an additional 25 minutes before drinking.

o Alternate method: Chlorine ampules
  - Fill your canteen with the cleanest water available.
  - Mix one ampule of chlorine with one-half canteen cup of water; stir the mixture with a clean device until contents are fully dissolved.
  - Pour one canteen capful of the above solution into your canteen of water.
  - Place the cap on your canteen and shake. Slightly loosen the cap and tip the canteen over to allow leakage around threads. Tighten cap and wait 30 minutes before drinking.
  - If the nuclear, biological, and chemical (NBC) canteen cap is used, then use two caps of the solution.

> **note**
>
> By wearing gloves or wrapping the chlorine ampule in paper or cloth, you can avoid cutting your hands when breaking open the glass ampule.

o Alternate method: Emergency water treatment kit (Chlor-Floc tablets)
  - Tear off the top of the plastic water treatment bag at the perforation (first-time use).
  - Fill the treatment bag one-half full with the cleanest water available; add 1 tablet.
  - Fold bag tightly three times and fold tabs in.
  - Hold bag firmly and shake until tablet dissolves. Swirl 10 seconds. Let the bag sit for 4 minutes. Swirl again for 10 seconds.
  - Let bag sit for an additional 15 minutes.
  - Insert filter pouch in neck of canteen. Pour water from bag through the filter into the canteen. Avoid pouring sediment into the filter.
  - Rinse the filter with treated water after use. Always filter through the same side of the filter.
  - Rinse sediment from treatment bag. Save bag for water treatment only.

> **CAUTION**
>
> Do not drink from the treatment bag! The water is still contaminated and must be filtered before drinking. Not filtering may cause stomach and intestinal disorders.

Table 5	Drops of Household Bleach to Be Added to a 1-Quart Canteen	
Available Chlorine	**Clean Water**	**Cold or Cloudy Water**
1%	10	20
4% to 6%	2	4
7% to 10%	1	2

○ Alternate method: Household bleach

note

Ensure that the bleach is unscented.

- Fill your canteen with the cleanest water possible.
- Read the label on the bleach bottle to determine the amount of available chlorine. Liquid chlorine laundry bleach usually has about 5% to 6% available chlorine. Based on the strength of the household bleach and the type of water (**Table 5**), add the chlorine to the canteen as directed in the next step.
- Place the cap on your canteen and shake. Slightly loosen the cap and tip the canteen over to allow leakage around threads. Tighten the cap and wait 30 minutes before drinking the water.

○ Alternative method: Boiling
- When chlorine or iodine is not available, bring water to a rolling boil for 5 minutes.
- In an emergency, boiling water for just 15 seconds will help.

note

Boiled water must be protected from recontamination.

CAUTION

If water is suspected of NBC contamination, do not attempt to treat it. Seek a quartermaster water supply.

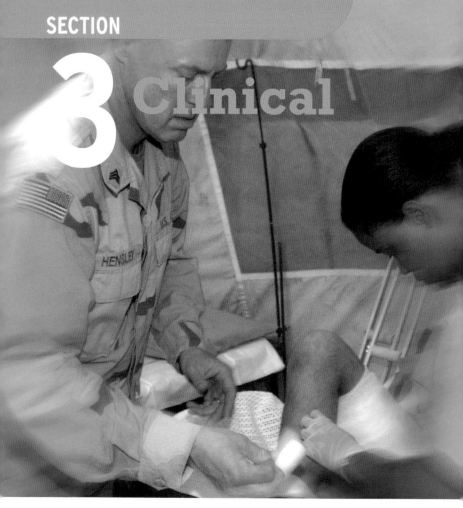

Patient Assessment

Scene Size-Up

① Take Basic Symptom Inventory (BSI). Make sure to wear gloves.

② Determine whether the scene is safe: Evaluate the scene regarding the safety of both the patient and emergency personnel.

③ Determine the mechanism of injury (MOI): Consider the mechanism of injury and what wounds and complications might arise from those injuries. This will guide the type of exam to be performed:

- Significant MOI = Rapid trauma assessment
- Nonsignificant MOI = Focused history and exam

4 Determine the number of patients: Depending on the number of patients, the severity of injuries, and estimated evacuation times, patients may need to be triaged, and resources may need to be reserved for the casualties with the greatest chance of survival.

5 Request additional help: Consider the need for additional help; this is usually based on the number of patients. The MOI may dictate additional personnel or equipment (e.g., additional ambulances, fire department with extraction equipment).

6 Consider stabilization of the spine: Evaluate the MOI and decide if C-spine and long spine stabilization and immobilization are warranted.

The Initial Assessment

The initial assessment of the patient consists of checking the ABCs (Airway, Breathing, and Circulation) and arriving at D (Decision regarding transport and type of examination). Look for and treat all life threats.

1 Formulate a general impression of the patient.

- Evaluate the casualty's appearance and condition using the power of observation. Look for clues to what happened (ties into MOI). *Think!*
- At a minimum, the evaluation should include the following: Patient's approximate age, weight, body position, and appearance (note any signs of distress); and whether any odors are present (e.g., alcohol, urine, vomit, or the fruity-smelling breath of diabetic ketoacidosis).

2 Gain C-spine control: It is a good idea to gain C-spine control prior to asking the patient any questions, because the patient may turn his or her head to answer you. If you have an assistant, that individual can help here.

3 Assess mental status: Determine level of consciousness (LOC) and responsiveness (AVPU).

- Examples: The patient's eyes are open and patient is moaning in pain; patient responded to me when I talked to him (AVPU evaluation). Patient is A&O $\times$ 3 = Alert and oriented (O) to person, place, and time.

Patient is A&O × 4 = Alert and oriented to person, place, and time, and patient knows exactly what happened to him.

o AVPU
- A = Alert
- V = responds to Verbal stimuli
- P = responds only to Painful stimuli
- U = Unresponsive to all stimuli

4 Determine chief complaint and apparent life threats: Ask the patient what happened, how it happened, where it hurts, when it happened, and so forth. If this information is written down, it should be in the patient's own words. Try to get basic patient information, such as name, age, and so forth.

5 Check the ABCs.

o A = Airway
- Check the airway for patency using appropriate methods (e.g., head-tilt with chin-lift or jaw thrust).
- Consider an airway adjunct. Insert a nasopharyngeal airway (NPA) or an oropharyngeal airway (OPA) and then reassess the airway immediately to determine if the airway is still patent (assess, treat, reassess).

o B = Breathing
- Is the patient breathing? Is ventilation adequate? (Rate should be 8 to 24, with adequate depth.)
- If the patient is not breathing (apneic), immediately begin assisting ventilations with a bag-valve-mask (BVM) device with supplemental oxygen (if available) before continuing the assessment.
- Assess adequacy of ventilation by putting your ear near the patient's mouth and looking toward the chest. Look, listen, and feel for air movement. Estimate the rate and depth of the patient's breaths.
  - If the patient is unresponsive with a breathing rate lower than 8 breaths/min, ventilate with BVM and 100% oxygen once every 5 seconds while still controlling the C-spine. This is also appropriate if the patient's breathing is faster than 8 breaths/min but inadequate in depth.
  - If the depth of ventilations is sufficient but the rate is faster than 24 breaths/min, administer high-concentration oxygen by nonrebreather mask.
  - If ventilations are determined to be adequate in rate and depth, you may proceed to assessing C (Circulation).

- If ventilations are determined to be inadequate once oxygen is applied, you must search for the cause of the inadequate ventilations by following the IAP (Inspect, Auscultate, Palpate) steps. The chest should be exposed and assessed for wounds, equal and bilateral expansion, and breathing quality; then auscultate the four fields and palpate the chest.
  - Inspection: Check for Deformities, Contusions, Abrasions, Punctures/Penetrations, Burns, Tenderness, Lacerations, Swelling (DCAP-BTLS).
  - Auscultation: Auscultate the four fields.
  - Palpation: Start with a "shoulder rock"—push on anterior chest/shoulders, breast line, and sides, feeling for Tenderness, Instability, Crepitus (TIC). Also check posterior chest (downside) from shoulder and lateral chest, feeling back until hands meet; then check the opposite side, and finally check under the small of the back.

note

If the patient is not breathing adequately for any reason, perform a complete assessment of the chest (IAP) in order to determine the nature of the inadequacy and perform any necessary treatment (in accordance with prehospital trauma life support [PHTLS]).

- C = Circulation
  - Two-step process: (1) Look for and treat life-threatening bleeding. (2) Check circulation: Start with radial pulses first; if absent, check for a carotid pulse. Then check skin temperature, color, and condition.
  - Step 1: Look and feel for hemorrhage with a blood sweep going from head to toe, pulling your hands out after each stroke and looking at them for the presence of blood (**Table 6**).
    - Start at the head and work your way down the body in a systematic way, being sure to get your hands all the way under each body part.
    - At the posterior of the chest, be sure to feel the whole back for possible wounds that can't be seen.
      - Technique: Feel the posterior chest (downside) by reaching under the shoulder with one hand and under the lateral side of the chest with the other, until your hands meet. Spread the fingers out and rake back, feeling for any wounds. Then check the opposite side in

the same manner. Next, move down the back, checking under the small of the back and then under the abdomen.
- At the pelvis, use the same technique as just described, but under the buttocks.
- Check each leg, including the bottom of the feet, and then check each arm and the hands.

note ———————————————————————

Control any hemorrhage as you find it. Use direct pressure, pressure dressings, elevation, pressure points, and even tourniquets as needed.

———————————————————————

note ———————————————————————

If you are in the Care Under Fire phase of a combat environment, a tourniquet would be the most appropriate first measure to use to control extremity hemorrhage. This may be loosened in the Tactical Care phase while other methods are used to control hemorrhage.

———————————————————————

■ Step 2: Check circulation.
- Check radial pulses first. If radial pulses are absent, then check for a carotid pulse; if that is absent, begin CPR.
- Check the skin temperature, color, and condition.

note ———————————————————————

Checking the pulses starting with the radials and then carotids can also serve as a quick check of the patient's blood pressure. A radial pulse represents a systolic blood pressure (BP) of at least 80 mm Hg, while carotids would represent a systolic BP of only about 60 mm Hg.

———————————————————————

Radial pulse:	Pressure ≥ 80 mm Hg
Femoral pulse:	Pressure ≥ 70 mm Hg
Carotid pulse:	Pressure ≥ 60 mm Hg

6 D = Decision and Determine priority (the transport decision)

○ This is the final step of the initial assessment.
○ The transport decision and type of exam (i.e., a focused exam for a specific injury or a rapid trauma assessment for more traumatic MOIs and

Table 6 Hemorrhage Classification

Hemorrhage Classification	Class I	Class II	Class III	Class IV
Blood loss (mL)	Up to 750	750-1500	1500-2000	>2000
Blood loss (% blood volume)	Up to 15%	15-30%	30-40%	>40%
Pulse rate	<100	>100	>120	>140
Blood pressure	Normal	Normal	Decreased	Decreased
Pulse pressure (mm Hg)	Normal or increased	Decreased	Decreased	Decreased
Capillary blanch test	Normal	Positive	Positive	Positive
Respiratory rate	14-20	20-30	30-40	>35
Urine output (mL/hr)	>30	20-30	5-15	Negligible
CNS/Mental status	Slightly anxious	Mildly anxious	Anxious and confused	Confused and lethargic
Fluid replacement (3:1 rule)	Crystalloid	Crystalloid	Crystalloids and Blood	Crystalloids and Blood

critical injuries) is decided now. You should be developing run-sheet, Field Medical Card, and/or MEDEVAC request information in your head or assigning an assistant to write it down.

The Rapid Trauma Assessment

1 E = Expose/Evaluate (rapid trauma assessment)

○ Expose areas as necessary: "You can't treat what you can't see." Be aware of environmental conditions and protect the patient from exposure to the elements; provide some level of dignity for the patient as well.

○ Inspect all body parts for DCAP-BTLS, looking for any life-threatening injuries not identified in the initial assessment.

■ Head: Inspect for DCAP-BTLS.

■ Neck: The neck should be inspected and palpated. Look for the possibility of airway compromise from a laceration or puncture into the trachea. Also, the neck should be assessed for tracheal deviation and jugular vein distention (JVD).

• Apply a C-collar if indicated by MOI. If significant MOI, in-line stabilization must be maintained until the patient is properly secured to a backboard.

- Chest: Reassess the chest using IAP (Inspection, Auscultation, Palpation). The chest should be exposed and assessed for wounds, equal bilateral expansion, and breathing rhythm and quality. Auscultate the four chest fields and palpate the chest looking for TIC.
  - Inspection: Perform a more detailed inspection and re-inspect the chest for bilateral equality of expansion. Recheck any treatments already applied (e.g., occlusive dressings).
  - Auscultation: Auscultate the four chest fields.
  - Palpation (*Note:* If already done in the initial assessment, then it can be skipped here.)
    - Palpate the thorax for TIC.
    - Start with the patient's clavicles and shoulders, pressing down slowly but firmly. Palpate down both sides of the patient's chest wall simultaneously, pushing from front to back and from right side to left side.
    - The exam should proceed in a systematic order that covers all areas of the chest.
    - Re-inspect the posterior chest (downside) if treatments were applied in initial assessment (e.g., occlusive dressing).
- Abdomen: Inspect and palpate for DCAP-BTLS, and more specifically for TRD-P (Tenderness, Rigidity, Distention, and Pulsating masses).
- Pelvis: Inspect and palpate for DCAP-BTLS and TIC.
  - Visually inspect for deformities, contusions/bruising, incontinence, priapism, and blood from the genital area or rectum.
  - Palpate for tenderness, instability, and crepitus by a pelvic rock and pushing on the symphysis pubis (if there are no signs or symptoms of a fracture). Do not palpate for crepitus if you suspect a pelvic fracture. If you suspect a fracture, then treat it as such. Only palpate for crepitus in the pelvis once. *Remember:* Pelvic palpation should only be done in the absence of any other signs and/or symptoms (S/S) of a fracture.
  - If patient is awake and complaining of pelvic pain or if you see any S/S of a pelvic fracture, do not palpate the pelvis. If in doubt, consider the pelvis fractured and treat it as such.
- Lower extremities: Examine the legs and feet looking for DCAP-BTLS. Reassess any bandages already applied, and expose any areas not yet checked. Check PMS (Pulse/Motor/Sensory).
- Upper extremities: Examine the upper extremities looking for DCAP-BTLS. Reassess any bandages and reinforce them if necessary. Check PMS.

- Posterior: Set up the stretcher prior to checking the posterior. Logroll the patient with good cervical and long spine control, inspect the posterior chest for wounds, and if necessary apply or reinforce any dressings. Sweep the back of the legs, buttocks, back, and the back of the head looking for DCAP-BTLS. Palpate ("walk") the long spine from the sacrum to T1 or the bottom of the C-collar looking for step-offs, deviations, and deformities. Then carefully roll the patient on the stretcher.

> **note**
>
> Remember, if a pelvic fracture is suspected, you should not logroll the patient. Instead, use a scoop stretcher and check as much of the posterior as possible through the space in the scoop stretcher, using the local protocol.

- Immediately reassess ABCs: After the logroll, do a check of the ABCs and any treatments that have been applied to the patient thus far, such as bandages, that might have come loose during the logroll.
- Secure the patient to the stretcher.

> **note**
>
> It is never wrong to recheck ABCs. When you logroll or move a patient, things might fall off (bandages, tubes, IVs, etc.) Reassess after any move!

2 F = Full set of vitals and SAMPLE history

○ SAMPLE history (can be gathered as the soldier medic works throughout the initial assessment)
  - S = Signs and symptoms
  - A = Allergies
  - M = Medications
  - P = Prior medical history of significance
  - L = Last meal
  - E = Events leading up to the injury

3 G = Get out (load the patient in the ambulance and transport)

○ Move the patient to the evacuation vehicle after stabilization.
○ Call report into the receiving hospital or next echelon.

> **note**
>
> When moving the patient to the ambulance, the senior combat medic should be at the patient's head (i.e., at the head of the stretcher) so he or she can monitor the patient while moving. The patient's feet should be pointed in the direction of travel.

Detailed Physical Exam

o H = "Head to toe—treat as you go" = Detailed physical exam.

o All life threats should already have been managed by this point. This is where the medic can tie up loose ends, such as treating minor wounds and non-life-threatening injuries, reinforcing bandages, and applying splints. This can all be done in the evacuation vehicle or while waiting for air evac to arrive. If air evac arrives early or you quickly reach the next echelon, the patient can be transferred even though the detailed physical exam is not complete (because all the major wounds and injuries have been stabilized prior to this point).

  ■ Always start by reassessing the patient's ABCs. Remember that while performing an ongoing patient assessment, you should reassess your patient's ABCs and vitals every 5 to 15 minutes depending on the patient's condition.

  ■ Inspect all areas for DCAP-BTLS.

  > **note**
  >
  > In the detailed exam the only additional items inspected are the face, eyes, ears, nose, and mouth.

o Head (HEENT): Check eyes for DCAP-BTLS, discoloration, and foreign bodies; blood in anterior chamber; and pupil size, equality, and reaction to light. Look in the ears, nose, mouth, and throat for trauma and bleeding; at the same time, check the airway again for patency.

o Neck: Reassess DCAP-BTLS, tracheal deviation, and jugular vein distention (it will be limited by C-collar).

o Chest: Re-inspect the chest (IAP) just as in the rapid trauma assessment, but in more detail. Inspect again and check any dressings already applied. Re-auscultate the lungs; the patient's condition can change over time. Palpate again, in a more detailed fashion, looking for TIC and DCAP-BTLS.

- Abdomen: Inspect and palpate for DCAP-BTLS, and more specifically for TRD-P (Tenderness, Rigidity, Distention, and Pulsating masses).
- Pelvis: Perform a more detailed exam, again looking for TIC and DCAP-BTLS.
- Lower extremities: Perform a more detailed exam and reassess bandages to lower extremities. Inspect for DCAP-BTLS any areas not checked yet. Check Pulse/Motor/Sensory (PMS).
- Upper extremities: Reassess and expose if necessary. Do a more detailed inspection for DCAP-BTLS. Check PMS.
- Posterior: Evaluate as much of the posterior body as you can reach for other injuries that may have been missed earlier. Simply reassess the flanks and as much of the spinal area as you can touch without moving the patient.

---

note

The posterior should be checked extremely well during the log-roll step because it is extremely difficult to check the back once the patient is secured to a backboard.

- Reassess ABCs, vitals, and disability every 5 minutes for critical patients and every 15 minutes for all others.

Documentation Using the SOAP Method

The SOAP method is the standard for documentation in medical treatment records and is designed to allow easy reference for follow-up care. The method follows the standard and natural flow of a patient interview, beginning with the Subjective data (S), proceeding to the Objective findings (O), arriving at an Assessment (A), and formulating a treatment Plan (P). Appropriate SOAP notes adhere to the guidelines presented here. Each complaint covered by this reference manual is presented using the SOAP method so as to allow the experienced medic to make detailed notes using the SOAP method and to assist the less experienced medic in providing adequate documentation.

- Subjective: This portion of the note includes all information of a historical nature; that is, what the patient tells you the trouble is, how long it has been bothering him or her, and other important parts of the patient's medical history. It should be noted that this portion of the patient interview may well be the most significant contribution in providing quality patient care. The existence of certain complaints, circumstances, or methods of injury can often lead the examiner to concentrate on a special part of the physical examination, and may greatly influence the final assessment and treatment plan. *Some subjective findings will require the patient to be referred to a medical officer.* An appropriate subjective note will contain the following information:

- Age
- Race
- Sex
- Chief complaint(s)
- Duration of chief complaint
- Circumstances surrounding onset of chief complaint
- Relevant past medical history
- Pertinent positives (e.g., vomiting, diarrhea, fever, etc.)
- Pertinent negatives (e.g., *no* vomiting, diarrhea, fever, etc.)
- Significant social habits (e.g., alcohol, tobacco, etc.)

note

A history of allergies to medications and current use of medication are also considered an important part of the subjective note but will be documented on the SF600 (Chronological Record of Medical Care). As part of the history interview, it is very important to include social habits. You should ask about alcohol consumption and document what kind of alcohol, how much is consumed, and when. A smoking history should be documented in pack years. You can calculate pack years by multiplying the number of cigarette packs smoked per day by the number of years the patient has smoked. For example, if a 30-year-old woman smokes two packs of cigarettes a day for 20 years, she would have a 40 pack year smoking history. Patients who chew tobacco should also have this history documented.

- An example of a good subjective history for a 21-year-old man who injured his right ankle would be as follows: 21 y/o male presents c/o of a sprained right ankle ×24 hours. Patient injured ankle yesterday while attempting a right PLF, heard a "snap" and can only ambulate with assistance; returned to his barracks hoping to "sleep it off" but decided to come in after his ankle swelled and turned blue.
- Objective: This portion of the note includes all the examiner's observations and physical findings. It may also include the results of pertinent

laboratory and x-ray studies. It must be realized that a medical record is a legal document and that good intentions don't make good medical notes. A basic rule of thumb to remember is that if you didn't do it, don't chart it. Likewise, remember that if it isn't charted, then legally you did not perform that part of the examination. An appropriate objective note will demonstrate that the care provider has performed at least those parts of the physical examination that are relevant to the chief complaint, and should adhere to the guidelines listed under each complaint in this manual. *Some objective findings will require the patient to be referred to a medical officer.* A complete objective note will contain the following information:

- General appearance
- Indications of obvious distress
- Pertinent physical examination findings
- Relevant laboratory results
- Relevant x-ray and/or imaging studies

○ Assessment: This portion of the note is frequently given the most attention and concern by many care providers and by most patients. It is, however, the least important in the process of providing safe, quality patient care. It should be remembered that what we label a disease or condition is nowhere near as important as the process of first recognizing the patient's problem and then ensuring that the problem is treated or referred in a timely and successful manner. This manual will generally provide the medic with the guidance necessary to reach a reasonable assessment. It is assumed that the art of arriving at more specific assessments will develop with experience. *Some assessments will require referral to a medical officer.*

○ Plan: This portion of the note includes all medications prescribed and treatments given; special instructions, diets, or physical limitations imposed; disposition; and plans for follow-up. Immediately following the plan should be the care provider's identification data, to including (either stamped or printed) the care provider's rank, name, military occupational specialty, Social Security number, and signature. *Many plans will require consultation with a medical officer.* An adequate plan will contain the following information:

- Medication (include strength, dosage schedule, and duration)
- Special instructions
- Disposition (duty, profile, quarters, referrals)
- Follow-up plans

Disposition and Referral

○ Profiles, quarters, and bedrest

- Unless specifically authorized by the supervising medical officer and local SOP, screeners are not authorized to issue profiles or quarters/bedrest. This manual may suggest certain periods of limited physical activity, or periods of quarters/bedrest. It is assumed that care providers will follow local SOP and consult with or refer to a medical officer when the plan section of this manual suggests a profile or quarters. Some helpful points to remember:

  - Profiles should be written in nonmedical language and should be specific concerning physical limitations.
  - Profiles should have a specific expiration date. For example: "No running until 15 April" or "Quarters for 24 hrs then return to base at 0630 on 15 April."
  - Profiles that contain such terms as "×14 hrs" or "×3 days" may be misunderstood, particularly if the patient was seen in the afternoon or on a Friday.
  - The term "quarters" means restriction and rest in the patient's place of domicile (e.g., barracks, BEQ, BOQ, etc.) and should allow the patient freedom of movement within his or her living space. In other words, the patient may be free to use the day room and so forth. Patients on quarters may not perform military duties.
  - The term "bedrest" means the patient is restricted to his or her bed, with allowances for necessary travel to the dining facility and latrine. Patients on bedrest may not perform any military duties.
  - *Patients ill or injured enough to be placed on bedrest or quarters require daily follow-up at the temporary mobilization center and/or battalion aid station* (TMC/BAS).
  - It should be remembered that profiles and duty limitations are only strong suggestions issued to command channels by medical authorities. Commanders may decide that the successful completion of a mission requires that a soldier "break" his or her profile. In such an instance, the commander takes responsibility for his or her actions. Medical personnel must continue to support and follow the concerned soldier's health.

○ Referral to supervising medical officer

- This manual sets forth many instances and circumstances in which referral to a medical officer is mandatory. Screeners should feel free and comfortable in seeking guidance from their physician's assistant (PA) or physician whenever doubt exists. ALL COMPLAINTS OR

CONDITIONS NOT COVERED IN THE COMPLAINT SECTION OF THIS MANUAL REQUIRE CONSULTATION WITH OR REFERRAL TO A MEDICAL OFFICER. Consult if you have *any* doubt.

- The requirements for referral *do not* imply that the screener must halt his or her evaluation of the patient immediately upon encountering a condition for referral. On the contrary, unless the patient's condition is emergent (significantly abnormal vital signs, altered mental status, severe pain or injury), the screener should continue to fully question and examine the patient to the best of his or her ability. After completing as much of the assessment as possible, the screener should present all of the findings, including the reason for consultation or referral to the supervising medical officer.

Complaints

Abdominal Pain

Abdominal pain is a common complaint, and although the most common causes in young adults are mild and self-limited, there are many serious considerations that must be ruled out. Such a large list is beyond the scope of this manual. The screener must, however, take a thorough history, and make referrals as appropriate. See the discussions on NAUSEA AND VOMITING and DIARRHEA AND CONSTIPATION as a cross-reference.

1 Subjective

- General (quality, location, onset, duration, radiation of pain)
- Aggravating or mitigating factors
- Associated fever, diarrhea, constipation, nausea, vomiting, chest pain, or back pain
- History of trauma
- Appetite and last meal
- Medications, alcohol ingestion
- Past treatment or evaluation

2 Objective

- Vital signs, including postural blood pressure and pulse
- Sclera icterus, jaundice (appearance of mucus membranes)
- Sounds of lungs and heart (abnormal sounds)
- Appearance of abdomen (flat, protuberant, distended)
- Bowel sounds (normal, increased, or deceased)
- Tenderness, masses on abdominal palpation

- Guarding or rebound tenderness
- Psoas or obturator signs
- Costovertebral angle (CVA) tenderness
- Hernia (males)
- Guaiac-positive stool, any pain during rectal examination

3 Assessment

- Acute gastroenteritis: Pain is usually mild, crampy, and poorly localized, with nausea, vomiting, and diarrhea. See discussion on NAUSEA AND VOMITING.
- Heartburn or gastroesophageal reflux (GER): Mild epigastric, substernal burning sensation, usually after meals. Relieved by antacids.
- Pain from abdominal muscle stress: Excessive coughing or vomiting causes diffuse abdominal wall discomfort. Afebrile; may have minimal diffuse guarding.
- Hepatitis: Malaise, nausea, right upper quadrant (RUQ) pain and tenderness, jaundice, dark urine.
- Abdominal emergency: Severe abdominal pain, vomiting blood, bloody stools, high fever, rigid abdomen, positive heel tap, inability to stand or sit straight without pain.
- Appendicitis: Gradual onset of diffuse pain that migrates to right lower quadrant (RLQ). Fever usually less than 101°F (38.3°C) initially; RLQ and left lower quadrant (LLQ) rebound tenderness (Rovsing's sign). Psoas and obturator signs are positive if it is a retrocecal appendix. Elevated white blood count (WBC).
- Peptic ulcer: Burning, gnawing epigastric pain, often episodic 1 to 4 hours after meals. Relieved by food or antacids. Deep epigastric tenderness.
- Pelvic inflammatory disease (PID): Progressive lower abdominal pain, cramping, and fever in females. Adnexal tenderness on pelvic examination. (Do not perform a pelvic exam unless under the direct supervision of a medical officer.)

4 Plan

- Acute gastroenteritis is usually self-limited. Treat with clear liquid diet, rest, and acetaminophen (Tylenol). Kaopectate or Donnagel may be given for diarrhea.
- Heartburn usually responds well to antacids such as Gaviscon or Mylanta. Recurrent episodes may indicate underlying ulcer or reflux.
- For pain from abdominal stress, reassure the patient that there is no evidence of serious organic disease. Tylenol, antacids, and rest help the pain.

5 Medical officer consultation is required in the following cases:

- Severe or recurrent abdominal pain
- Severe nausea or vomiting
- Bloody, coffee-ground vomitus
- Bloody, tarry stools
- Fever greater than 100°F (37.8°C)
- Jaundice, icterus
- Postural vital signs (BP drops more than 10 mm Hg systolic and pulse rises higher than 20 beats/min after standing)
- Abdominal distention
- Absence of bowel sounds
- Moderate to severe tenderness or masses on palpation
- Guarding or rebound tenderness
- CVA tenderness
- Hernia
- Positive guaiac test
- When the screener is in doubt or uncomfortable with the case

Acne

Acne is a very common skin condition of adolescents and young adults. It is a result of hormonal influences increasing the activity of the oil glands. In women, acne may be worse during the menstrual cycle.

1 Subjective

- Age at onset
- Previous treatment
- Relationship to menstrual cycle in women
- Cammo face paint, oily hair preparations, and cosmetic use

2 Objective

- Distribution
- Comedones (blackheads)
- Papulopustular lesions
- Cystic lesions
- Scarring

3 Assessment
Acne may be graded as follows:

- Grade I is usually limited to the facial area and is characterized by comedones and few papular lesions. Scarring is not present.
- Grade II consists of comedones, a moderate amount of inflamed papules, and occasional scarring.

- Grade III has the lesions described above plus pustules; papulopustular formation is moderate, and scarring is seen.
- Grade IV is the most severe form. In addition to the lesions above, cystic lesions are present. Scarring may be severe.

4 Plan

- Grade I may be treated with topical preparations containing benzoyl peroxide, and/or with tretinoin (Retin-A).
- Grades II and III are treated with the topical agents listed for grade I, but tetracycline PO is added.
- Grade IV requires referral to a dermatologist for more intensive therapy.
- All patients must be instructed to avoid picking or squeezing lesions, to avoid the use of oily cosmetics, and to practice meticulous cleansing of the face and affected areas.

5 Medical officer consultation is required in the following cases:

- Grade II or III acne (antibiotics will be required)
- Grade IV acne (a referral to dermatology will be required)
- When the screener is in doubt or is uncomfortable with the case

Allergies and Hay Fever

Patients with allergies often have family histories of multiple allergic disorders, including hay fever, asthma, and eczema.

1 Subjective

- Onset and duration of symptoms
- Previous occurrences
- Known allergies; exposure to known allergens
- Sneezing
- Runny, stuffy nose
- Eye irritation
- Shortness of breath, wheezing
- Current/previous medications
- Family history of allergic conditions

2 Objective

- Temperature
- Able to touch chin to chest without pain
- Conjunctival injection, lacrimation
- Nasal discharge; pale, boggy, edematous nasal turbinates
- Wheezing, increased rate of respirations, stridor

3 Assessment

○ Allergic conjunctivitis: Conjunctiva injected with increased lacrimation, itching, and sneezing.
○ Allergic rhinitis: Nonpurulent nasal discharge with associated sneezing.
○ Hay fever: Eye and nasal signs present with occasional wheezing. Allergies during spring are usually due to tree pollens; during the summer, to grass pollens; and during the fall, to weed pollens, but fungus spores may also cause hay fever symptoms.

4 Plan: The best treatment is identification and avoidance of the offending allergen, but the systemic effects can be treated symptomatically with antihistamines. If eye irritation is significant, add Visine. If nasal congestion is severe, nasal spray or drops containing phenylephrine (Neo-Synephrine) may also be used for periods not to exceed 3 days.

5 Medical officer consultation is indicated for the following cases:

○ Pain when touching chin to chest
○ Fever greater than 100°F (37.8°C)
○ Purulent nasal discharge
○ Shortness of breath, stridor
○ When simple antihistamines have not been effective
○ When the screener is in doubt or uncomfortable with the case

Ankle Sprain

Ankle sprains are common in the active duty population due to the increased level of physical activity. Ankle sprains can be grouped as grade I simple sprains, or as grade II or grade III sprains, which are significant. Fractures are frequently associated with significant sprains.

1 Subjective

○ Mechanism of injury, position of foot at time of injury (inverted, supinated)
○ Time of occurrence
○ Past trauma
○ Pain or discomfort

2 Objective

○ Inability to bear weight
○ Swelling (edema)

- Ecchymosis
- Localization of tenderness, pain (medial or lateral malleolus, anterior joint margin)
- Range of motion (ROM), passive and active
- Stability, drawer sign
- Distal neurovascular exam (sensation, pulses, capillary refill)
- X-ray results, if indicated

3 Assessment

- Grade I sprain: Antalgic gait. Able to bear weight. Minimal, if any, edema; no ecchymosis; mild tenderness of either malleolar area; no drawer sign; neurovascular status and ROM intact.
- Grade II sprain: Unable to bear weight. Edema; possible ecchymosis; acute tenderness; no drawer sign; neurovascular status intact; ROM reduced. An x-ray should be done to rule out an associated fracture.
- Grade III sprain: Unable to bear weight. Edema, ecchymosis present; acute tenderness; positive drawer sign; ROM markedly decreased; instability present; neurovascular status may be compromised. An x-ray is necessary to rule out an associated fracture.

4 Plan

- Grade I sprains are initially treated with ice, compression, and elevation for 24 to 48 hours. Crutches are indicated for up to 48 hours in grade I sprains. Anti-inflammatory agents (e.g., Motrin) and ace wrap protection are indicated for 5 to 7 days, with gradually increased exercises.
- Grade II sprains may require posterior or "U" splinting for 3 to 5 days with ice, elevation, crutches, and analgesics (Motrin). An ace wrap is indicated, with gradual increase of activity after 72 to 96 hours.
- Grade III sprains are a significant injury and will require immobilization using either a splint or non-weight-bearing cast. Initially, ice, compression, and elevation are used to reduce edema and pain. Crutches (without weight bearing) and follow-up with podiatry or orthopedics are usually indicated. Nonsteroidal anti-inflammatory drugs with a mild narcotic will often be needed for pain relief.
- In all sprains, physical activity must be reduced appropriately; this limitation will vary in length from 72 hours to several weeks.

5 Medical officer consultation is required in the following cases:

- Unable to bear weight
- Ecchymosis present

- Severe pain
- Loss of ROM
- Instability (positive drawer sign)
- When the screener is in doubt or uncomfortable with the case

Chest Pain

Chest pain offers a diagnostic challenge to the screener as well as to the PA or physician. Most chest pain among healthy soldiers is noncardiac in origin, but care must be taken to rule out heart disease in every case. Gastrointestinal, pulmonary, musculoskeletal, neurologic, and psychogenic problems can cause chest pain. The best way to differentiate these noncardiac from cardiac problems is to obtain a good history. A description of the pain is extremely important.

 Subjective

- Onset of pain
- Precipitating factor(s) of pain
- Duration of pain
- Predictable relief of pain
- Location of pain
- Quality of pain
- Pain intensity changing with respiration
- Previous episodes of pain
- Previous heart disease
- Nausea, vomiting, diaphoresis, shortness of breath (SOB)
- Fainting spells
- Trauma to chest wall
- Cough, fever
- Family history of heart disease
- Cardiac risk factors (smoker, hypertension, cholesterolemia, diabetes, sedentary lifestyle, abnormal ECG)

 Objective

- Elevated BP
- Tachycardic or irregular pulse
- Tenderness with palpation over area of chest pain
- Cyanosis
- Wheezing, rales
- Cardiac or pulmonary friction rub on inspiration
- Abnormal heart sounds
- Levine's sign (clutching fist to chest)

❸ Assessment: The main objective is to separate noncardiac from cardiac pain.

○ Cardiac pain, caused by insufficient blood to the heart muscle (ischemia), is called angina.

○ If the history reveals that the pain is induced by bending forward, touching the chest wall, breathing, or positioning of the body or arms, then it is highly unlikely that the pain is of cardiac origin.

○ If the pain lasts only a second or is constant over hours or days, then the pain is not due to angina.

○ If the pain is brought on immediately while lying down, again the pain is not due to angina.

○ Tenderness to palpation of the chest wall or pain in the chest wall with twisting of the upper body with otherwise negative findings indicates musculoskeletal pain (costochondritis).

○ Chest wall pain in large-breasted women may be due to inadequate breast support during exercise.

❹ Plan: Except in those instances where chest wall pain can be determined to be the cause, chest pain should be evaluated by a PA or physician. For chest wall pain, anti-inflammatory analgesics such as aspirin or Motrin (consult required) should be provided.

❺ Medical officer consultation is required in the following cases:

○ For all chest pain other than chest wall tenderness
○ When the screener is in doubt or uncomfortable with the case

Corns and Calluses

Corns and calluses develop in response to abnormal pressures against the skin of the foot. External pressure due to improper shoe wear and/or internal pressure from abnormal bony protuberances will frequently lead to the production of thickened, painful, hard skin over the bony prominence. In areas where moisture and perspiration collect, the skin becomes macerated and a soft corn develops.

❶ Subjective

○ Location
○ Duration
○ Pain
○ Aggravating and relieving factors

2 Objective

o Appearance
o Inspection of foot gear
o Signs of inflammation or infection
o Pain with direct or lateral pressure

3 Assessment

o Callus formation normally occurs over weight-bearing surfaces and consists of thickened, tender, hard skin. Margins often blend into the surrounding skin.
o Hard corns are usually found on the dorsal lateral aspect of the proximal interphalangeal (PIP) joint of the fifth toe. They are painful with direct pressure.
o Soft corns are most common in the fourth interdigital space.
o Plantar warts may be confused with calluses or corns. They generally have a central punctate area with surrounding thickened skin. Plantar warts are painful with lateral pressure and have punctate bleeding points when shaved.

4 Plan

o Removal of the external pressure is essential. Pads are helpful in blocking direct contact and reducing pressure on the corn or callus.
o Warm, soapy-water soaks followed by salicylic acid plaster or cream application will help eliminate the corn or callus.
o Corns and calluses may be treated by the patient using commercially available pumice stone.
o Corns and calluses may be shaved in thin layers to reduce discomfort.

5 Medical officer consultation is required in the following cases:

o Acute pain with weight bearing
o Inflammation or infection present
o Punctate bleeding points exposed when callus is trimmed
o When the screener is in doubt or uncomfortable with the case

Crabs/Lice

The crab louse is a tiny insect that lives only on humans, almost exclusively on the moist, hairy areas of the body—the groin and axillae. Sexual contact accounts for 99% of the transmission. Shared towels, linens, or underwear may rarely transmit the louse. Lice die rapidly when removed from their human host; they do not hide in the latrines or jump from bunk to bunk. They may be seen with the naked eye on skin or hair and appear about the size of a pinhead. Because their life cycle takes 2 to 3 weeks, it may take as long as 4 to 6 weeks before the crab population is large enough for the patient to notice the infestation. Use SEXUALLY TRANSMITTED DISEASES as a cross-reference.

1 Subjective

- Mild to moderate pubic or perianal itching
- Crabs noted by patient
- Rash
- Last sexual contact (LSC)

2 Objective

- Insects on skin or hair
- Egg cases (nits) attached to hair
- Above confirmed under microscope, if necessary
- Mild erythema of skin around insect (bite marks)

3 Assessment

- Crabs (pubic lice): Consistent with the above symptoms and signs. Vigorous scratching may result in secondary infection.
- Scabies: This is an infestation by the scabies mite, which is smaller than the crab louse and burrows into the skin. Scabies is not limited to the pubic region but spreads everywhere except the scalp, causing a very itchy rash.

4 Plan

- Crabs: Apply a lindane cream or lotion (such as Kwell) from the umbilicus to the knees, as well as to the armpits, if those are involved. This should be left on for 8 to 12 hours, then washed off. Permethrin (Rid) may be used as an alternate to Kwell. Very hairy individuals may have to apply these lotions from the neck down. A repeat application in 1 week is recommended.
- Scabies: Apply a lindane cream or lotion (such as Kwell) from the neck down, including the arms, for 8 to 12 hours, then wash off. Repeat application is usually not necessary.
- All bedding and clothing to be used within the next 30 days must be washed thoroughly in hot, soapy water, or dry cleaned. If hot water is unavailable, a disinfectant may be added to the wash. Laundering of clothes is to be done during the 12-hour treatment period.
- Patients must be cautioned to follow instructions carefully to avoid lindane skin reactions.

5 Medical officer consultation is required in the following cases:

○ Suspected scabies
○ Secondary infection
○ When the screener is in doubt or is uncomfortable with the case

Diarrhea and Constipation

Diarrhea and constipation are symptoms whose causes are usually acute and self-limited. In all cases it is important to obtain a detailed description of the patient's symptoms. Acute diarrhea implies frequent, watery bowel movements, not just loose stools. A dietary history can usually explain most cases of constipation and loose stools in young adults. The discussions on ABDOMINAL PAIN and NAUSEA AND VOMITING should be used as cross-reference.

1 Subjective

○ General (onset, frequency, amount, last bowel movement, color, consistency, odor, any recent changes)
○ Associated abdominal pain, painful bowel movements, fever, weight loss, flatulence, anxiety, lack of energy
○ Bloody or tarry (black) stools
○ Postural hypotension (the feeling as if one will faint upon arising suddenly)
○ Current medications (laxatives, antibiotics, codeine, antacids)
○ Appetite, last meal, current fluid consumption
○ Dietary history (dairy or meat products, fruit, fiber)
○ Recent travel to rural areas, tropics, or Third World countries
○ Prior evaluation or treatment

2 Objective

○ Vital signs, including postural blood pressure and pulse
○ Weight (if symptoms chronic)
○ Signs of viral upper respiratory infection (URI) on HEENT exam
○ Appearance of abdomen (flat, protuberant, distended)
○ Bowel sounds (normal, increased, decreased)
○ Tenderness on abdominal palpation
○ Guarding or rebound tenderness
○ Guaiac results on any stool; save specimen for possible microscopic examination for white blood cells (WBCs)

3 Assessment

○ Acute constipation: Usually situational, secondary to voluntary restraint, decreased intake, or rectal pain (hemorrhoids).

○ Chronic constipation: Usually due to a low-fiber, high-fat, high-carbohydrate diet, possibly exacerbated by laxative abuse. Flatulence and mild abdominal pain may also be observed.

○ Acute gastroenteritis: Diarrhea will be moderate and with acute onset, frequently with nausea, vomiting, malaise, and mild fever; occasionally with URI signs. Active bowel sounds and little, if any, abdominal tenderness.

○ Food poisoning: Similar to gastroenteritis. Bacterial toxins (e.g., staphylococci) often produce sudden onset of nausea and vomiting followed by diarrhea. Bacterial infections (e.g., salmonellae) usually produce only diarrhea of sudden onset. Clusters of cases with similar food histories are frequently seen.

○ Dysentery: Acute to subacute diarrhea with pus, mucus, and blood in stools; fever, malaise, and abdominal pain are observed. Stool positive for many WBCs.

○ Irritable bowel syndrome: Though common, it is a diagnosis made only when others have been excluded. Chronic, recurrent abdominal discomfort and flatulence, aggravated by anxiety and stress; diarrhea often alternates with constipation. Exam is usually normal.

○ Inflammatory bowel disease: Recurrent diarrhea, often mixed with blood, and worse at night; mild to moderate abdominal pain with accompanying weight loss.

4 Plan

○ Acute constipation responds well to laxatives, such as milk of magnesia. Stool softeners (e.g., Colace, Surfak) are helpful when painful bowel movements are part of the problem. Warm prune juice works wonders in relieving constipation. Try this first before giving out laxatives.

○ Chronic constipation should be treated with dietary modifications to increase the amount of fruit and fiber eaten. Bulk-forming agents (e.g., Metamucil) may be helpful, but laxatives are to be avoided.

○ Acute gastroenteritis is usually self-limited. Treat with a clear liquid diet, rest, and acetaminophen (Tylenol). Kaopectate or Donnagel may be given for diarrhea.

○ Food poisoning: If mild, treat like gastroenteritis. Report clusters of cases to Preventive Medicine.

○ Loose stools, without other symptoms, may be treated with Kaopectate.

○ Be sure to tell the patient to return for follow-up if the diarrhea persists longer than 48 hours or if he or she develops a fever.

⑤ Medical officer consultation is required in the following cases:

- Severe or recurrent diarrhea
- Severe or persistent abdominal pain
- Bloody, tarry stools
- Diarrhea of more than 48 hours duration
- Fever greater than 100°F (37.8°C)
- Postural vital signs (BP drops more than 10 mm Hg systolic, pulse rises more than 20 beats/min after standing)
- Abdominal distention
- Absence of bowel sounds
- Moderate to severe tenderness or masses on palpation
- Guarding or rebound tenderness
- Positive guaiac test
- When the screener is in doubt or uncomfortable with the case

Ear Pain, Drainage, or Sense of Fullness

Ear pain may be caused by an infection of the external canal, a middle ear infection, or eustachian tube dysfunction. It may be accompanied by tinnitus or decreased hearing.

① Subjective

- Pain in affected ear
- Associated URI symptoms
- Decreased hearing
- Trauma
- Drainage

② Objective

- Movement of pinna causes pain
- Tympanic membrane dull, retracted, hyperemic, or bulging
- External canal abraded or inflamed
- Temperature greater than 100°F (37.8°C)
- Cervical adenopathy
- Perforation
- Unable to see tympanic membrane due to cerumen
- Valsalva maneuver or pneumatic otoscopy

③ Assessment

- An external canal that is abraded or inflamed, with movement of the pinna causing pain, is consistent with external otitis.
- A dull, retracted drum is consistent with eustachian tube dysfunction.

- A hyperemic, bulging tympanic membrane is consistent with acute otitis media.
- A dull tympanic membrane behind which a fluid level with occasional air bubbles can be seen is consistent with serous otitis media.
- Ear pain and decreased hearing can result from hard impacted cerumen. In this case the tympanic membrane cannot be seen due to obstruction.

4 Plan

- External otitis is usually quite adequately treated with Domeboro otic solution. Occasionally an antibiotic-steroid combination may be required. In this case, medical officer consultation is required.
- Eustachian tube dysfunction is treated with decongestants and having the patient perform Valsalva maneuvers periodically.
- Acute otitis media usually requires antibiotics; therefore, medical officer consultation is required.
- Serous otitis media is treated in the same manner as eustachian tube dysfunction.
- A perforation of the tympanic membrane requires medical officer referral.
- Impacted cerumen can be removed by irrigation or carbamide peroxide (Debrox) solution. Curetting should only be done by the medical officer. Prior to irrigation, triethanolamine polypeptide oleate-condensate (Cerumenex) or carbamide peroxide (Debrox) should be placed in the affected ear and allowed to soften the cerumen for approximately 15 minutes. Prior to irrigation, make sure there is no perforation.

5 Medical officer consultation is required in the following cases:

- Trauma
- Temperature greater than 100°F (37.8°C)
- Perforation
- Hyperemic, bulging tympanic membrane
- When the screener is in doubt or is uncomfortable with the case

Fatigue

Fatigue is one of the most common symptoms for which adult patients seek medical attention. It may be described as a general tiredness, lack of energy, weariness, or a subjective sense of weakness and is often accompanied by a strong desire to sleep. Fatigue is normal when it is the result of a full day's work or sustained physical activity. Chronic fatigue, however, is not normal. The screener's objective is to separate normal individuals from those with significant anxiety, depression, or organic illness.

1 Subjective

- General (onset, duration, character of fatigue)
- Associated fever, loss of appetite, weight loss, headache, sore throat, muscle aches, or joint pains
- Sleep patterns (insomnia, early awakening)
- Anxiety (current stressful situations)
- Depression (feeling blue, loss of interest)
- Medications (sedatives, antihistamines, antidepressants)
- Living conditions—what is used for heat (wood, coal, gas, etc.)?
- Do other people in the household have the same complaint?

2 Objective

- Vital signs
- Appearance of patient (sick, tired, depressed)
- Pale skin, nailbeds, or mucosa
- HEENT exam (erythema of the throat)
- Lymphadenopathy (swollen, tender lymph nodes)
- Lungs (rales, wheezes)
- Heart (irregular rhythm, murmur, gallop, or rub)
- Abdomen (masses, tenderness)
- Hematocrit test results, if indicated

3 Assessment

- Normal tiredness: History of sustained hard work or physical activity without anxiety, depression, or trouble sleeping. Normal exam.
- Anxiety state: History of recent stressful situations, difficulty sleeping; fatigue lessens during day; mild headache may be present. Patient may appear anxious; exam is otherwise normal.
- Dysthymia: No set pattern, but usually accompanied by difficulty sleeping. Patient may appear depressed; physical exam is otherwise normal.
- Mononucleosis: Mild sore throat, fever; fatigue is relieved by rest. Exam reveals pharyngitis, cervical adenopathy. Positive mono spot test.
- Anemia: Patient usually complains lack of energy with physical activity, relieved by rest. Exam reveals pale nailbeds, skin, or mucosa; increased pulse. Anemia is seen with a hematocrit less than 43% in males, 38% in females.
- Chronic illness: Fatigue relieved by rest or decreased activity; muscle aches or joint pains, low-grade fever, and weight loss may also

be present. Exam may reveal lymphadenopathy or cardiac, lung, or abdominal abnormalities.

○ Carbon monoxide poisoning: Usually a normal exam; may see pale or bluish hue to nails. Will generally have a history of wood-, oil-, or coal-burning stove in a trailer, with other people in the household having the same complaint.

4 Plan

○ Patients with normal fatigue need reassurance that there is no evidence of underlying disease, and should be counseled to make maximum use of the sleeping time available to them.

○ Those with mild situational anxiety or dysthymia may only require reassurance that there is no evidence of underlying organic disease and that their symptoms are situational in origin. They should be instructed to return for follow-up if there is no improvement within 72 hours.

5 Medical officer consultation is required in the following cases:

○ Fever greater than 100°F (37.8°C)
○ Pulse greater than 100 beats/min at rest
○ Worsening symptoms over 2 weeks
○ History of greater than 5-pound weight loss in past month
○ Marked anxiety or depression
○ Inability to sleep
○ Pale nailbeds, skin, or mucosa
○ Adenopathy other than mild cervical adenopathy
○ Persistent joint or extremity pain
○ Abnormal lung, cardiac, or abdominal exam
○ Hematocrit below 42% in males, 38% in females
○ When the screener is in doubt or uncomfortable with the case

Friction Blisters

A blister will present as a bulla that may or may not be intact. Blisters are caused by mechanical friction. Blisters on the feet are usually a result of poorly fitted footwear.

 Subjective

○ General (location, onset, duration)
○ Pain
○ Activity limitations

2 Objective

- Appearance of lesions (location, solitary, multiple, intact, weeping)
- Signs of infection (warmth, erythema, pus)
- Gait, if blisters are on feet (observe whether patient is able to bear weight)

3 Assessment: Based on observation.

4 Plan

- Intact bullae are aspirated with a sterile needle and syringe after cleaning the area with povidone-iodine (Betadine). The skin is not debrided. The area is painted with tincture of benzoin twice. A dry dressing is applied. Soft shoes or duty limitations are not usually necessary, but may be indicated for 24 hours if the patient has difficulty bearing weight or walking.
- Bullae that have broken are cleaned with Betadine. The skin is preserved, and the area is painted with tincture of benzoin. A dry dressing is applied. Soft shoes or duty limitations are not usually necessary, but may be indicated for 24 hours if the patient has difficulty bearing weight or walking.

5 Medical officer consultation is required in the following cases:

- Extensive bullae formation
- Moderate to severe pain
- Infection
- When the screener is in doubt or uncomfortable with the case

Headaches

The majority of headaches are easily managed with simple medications. The onset of most headaches tends to be associated with stress, hangovers, or heat. The vast majority of these are "muscle tension" headaches. Vascular (migraine-type) headaches and headaches associated with febrile viral illnesses are also common in young adults.

1 Subjective

- Onset (gradual, sudden, awakens patient from sleep)
- Duration of the headache; are they recurrent?
- Location and character (unilateral, occipital, throbbing, band-like)
- Associated fever, loss of consciousness, nausea, vomiting, stiff neck, eye pain, visual changes, malaise
- Aggravating and/or mitigating factors

- Trauma within 72 hours
- Past treatment or evaluation

2 Objective

- Vital signs, especially temperature and blood pressure
- Able to touch chin to chest without pain
- HEENT exam (evidence of trauma, pupil size and reaction to light, sinus tenderness, tympanic membranes)
- URI signs
- Mental status (alert, oriented, drowsy, confused)

3 Assessment

- Simple headache usually has no specific physical findings.
- Musculoskeletal headache usually presents with a "squeezing band" encircling the head, and tightness of the neck muscles. It is usually bilateral and may continue for days.
- Migraine headaches are characterized by unilateral throbbing pain. There is usually nausea, vomiting, visual disturbances, and photophobia. Migraines generally have a history of recurrence.
- Fever accompanied by pain when performing the chin-to-chest maneuver suggests the possibility of meningitis. *Suspected meningitis is always an emergency!*

4 Plan

- Simple headaches are treated with analgesics, including acetaminophen (Tylenol) or aspirin.
- Musculoskeletal headaches can also be treated with analgesics, but moderate to severe headaches may require muscle relaxants.
- Migraine headaches will require specific antimigraine medications and probably temporary duty limitations.

5 Medical officer consultation is required in the following cases:

- Headaches associated with trauma, loss of consciousness, nausea and vomiting, or visual disturbances
- Increased blood pressure, temperature greater than 100°F (37.8°C)
- Inability to touch chin to chest without pain
- Moderate to severe musculoskeletal headaches
- Migraine-type headaches
- Inability to perform duty
- When the screener is in doubt or uncomfortable with the case

Hearing Loss

When a patient complains of hearing loss, the following examination should be done.

1 Subjective

- Onset
- Trauma
- Noise exposure
- URI symptoms
- Ear pain
- Affected ear(s)
- Current medications

2 Objective

- URI signs
- Perforation
- Otitis media
- Cerumen obstruction
- Audiometry screen

3 Assessment: If an obvious cause of hearing loss is not found, neurosensory hearing loss must be considered.

4 Plan: Hearing losses with no apparent cause must be referred to the medical officer for further evaluation. Other causes that are found on examination are treated as appropriate.

5 Medical officer consultation is required in the following cases:

- Audiogram shows a previously undocumented 10 dB loss at any frequency
- *No* apparent cause for the hearing loss
- Temperature greater than 100°F (37.8°C)
- Inflamed, bulging eardrum
- Perforation
- When the screener is in doubt or uncomfortable with the case

Hip Pain

Traumatic hip pain in young adults usually follows overuse (e.g., sports, running) or other strenuous physical activity. Hip fractures or dislocations in young adults with normal bones occur with high-energy trauma and are usually associated with other severe injuries.

1 Subjective

o Character of pain
o Onset/activity
o History of trauma or arthritis
o Involvement of other joints

2 Objective

o Palpable tenderness (exact location)
o ROM and associated pain
o Gait

3 Assessment

o Trochanteric bursitis: Usually presents with local pain over the greater trochanter with radiation down the lateral aspect of the thigh to the knee. Palpable tenderness is present. Internal rotation and abduction also causes pain.
o Tendonitis: Any of the muscles or tendons surrounding the hip joint may become strained and inflamed. Pain is localized to the affected part on palpation and is aggravated with motion.
o Slipped femoral epiphysis: A limp with hip pain develops. Usually seen in young males who are obese or tall and thin; rarely occurs over age 20. X-ray confirms diagnosis.

4 Plan

o Bursitis/tendonitis: Treatment consists of anti-inflammatory drugs, warm compresses, and reduction of aggravating factors until the patient is pain free.
o A slipped epiphysis will require an orthopedic consultation.

5 Medical officer consultation is required in the following cases:

o Inability to bear weight
o Decreased ROM
o Evidence of infection
o Crepitus present in joint with motion
o When the screener is in doubt or uncomfortable with the case

Hoarseness

The most common cause of hoarseness is acute laryngitis resulting from a viral infection. Other causes include bacterial infections, excessive use of the voice, allergic reactions, and inhalation of irritating substances.

1 Subjective

- Onset/precipitating factors
- Duration
- Associated symptoms (e.g., sore throat, cough, runny nose, muscle aches, hay fever)
- Pain with swallowing (dysphagia)
- Smoking history
- Contact with noxious substances

2 Objective

- Hoarse voice (aphonia)
- Temperature elevation
- Dyspnea
- Drooling
- Posterior oropharynx exam
- Throat culture results

3 Assessment: Based on subjective and objective findings. The key is to identify treatable causes.

4 Plan

- Viral laryngitis is self-limited, and no specific treatment is indicated. Some symptomatic relief may be gained with warm normal saline or hydrogen peroxide gargles or throat lozenges. Cepacol gargles or Chloraseptic may also be of benefit.
- Bacterial laryngitis is more frequently seen in children and is treated with appropriate antibiotics.
- Avoidance of irritating inhaled substances (e.g., tobacco smoke) should be stressed in those cases where this is the cause of the laryngitis.
- All patients with laryngitis should have voice rest and be advised to stop smoking, if applicable.
- Chronic hoarseness may be due to dysfunction of the vocal cords from tumor growth or neurologic deficit, and needs specialty care.

5 Medical officer consultation is required in the following cases:

- Pain with swallowing
- Temperature greater than 100°F (37.8°C)
- Dyspnea, drooling
- Positive culture for pathologic bacterial agent
- Symptoms present over 10 days
- When the screener is in doubt or is uncomfortable with the case

Knee Pain

Most unilateral knee pain is traumatic in origin. Acute trauma usually causes ligament sprains/strains or meniscal damage. Repeated mild trauma over long periods of time can lead to chondromalacia, chronic arthritis, or other problems.

1 Subjective

o History of knee "locking" or "giving way"
o History of trauma
o Prior knee surgery
o Precipitating factors
o Aggravating factors: deep knee bends, stair climbing
o Pain without weight bearing

2 Objective

o Discoloration (ecchymosis, erythema), swelling, deformity
o Effusion, crepitus
o Tenderness to palpation over joint line
o Warmth to touch
o Tenderness over medial/lateral collateral ligaments or menisci
o Patellar shift; tenderness with patellar compression
o Ligamentous instability with lateral and/or medial stress (lateral and/or medial collateral ligaments)
o Drawer sign; Lachman's sign (cruciate tear)
o McMurray's sign; Apley's sign (meniscal damage)
o Quadriceps symmetry (measured in centimeters)

3 Assessment

o Hot, tender knee with or without swelling may indicate intra-articular infection.
o Inability to fully extend knee and joint line tenderness may indicate meniscal injury.
o Tenderness over medial collateral ligaments (MCL) and/or lateral collateral ligaments (LCL) without laxity may indicate grade I sprain or strain.
o Mild laxity and tenderness of MCL/LCL indicate a possible grade II sprain.
o Ecchymosis and effusion present with laxity indicate a possible grade III sprain (torn ligament).
o A positive drawer sign or positive Lachman's sign indicates a probable cruciate injury.

- Patellar shift indicates possible patellar subluxation.
- Asymmetry of quadriceps, positive subpatellar crepitus, and pain while climbing stairs indicate possible chondromalacia.

4 Plan

- Grade I sprains: Initial treatment consists of ice packs, ace wrap, and elevation for the first 24 hours. Crutches may be indicated for comfort. Anti-inflammatory agents are used as required. Contusion without additional findings may also be treated with this plan.
- Chondromalacia, or retropatellar pain syndrome: Treated with quadriceps-strengthening exercises, the avoidance of deep knee bending, and nonsteroidal anti-inflammatory drugs (e.g., Motrin, Indocin).

5 Medical officer consultation is required in the following cases:

- Unable to bear weight
- Unable to fully extend leg
- History of knee "locking" or "giving way"
- Significant trauma
- Knee is warm, discolored, or deformed
- Effusion greater than 1 inch
- Ligamentous instability
- Positive drawer, Lachman's, or McMurray's sign
- When symptoms persist for more than 3 weeks
- When the screener is in doubt or uncomfortable with the case

Low Back Pain

Low back pain (LBP) is the leading "occupational" complaint in the United States. Common causes of LBP include unaccustomed physical activity, acute strain, and positional changes; in some cases, the cause is never determined. Most LBP is due to muscle strain, but a herniated intervertebral disc must always be ruled out.

1 Subjective

- General (location, onset, duration, nature, and intensity of pain)
- Radiation (does pain shoot down leg [sciatica], and if so, how far)
- Aggravating and/or relieving factors
- Weakness in legs
- Bowel/bladder dysfunction
- History of direct trauma to back
- Prior episodes of similar pain and prior evaluation

2 Objective

o Observe difficulty dressing or undressing
o Alignment, lordotic curve
o Palpation of spinous processes and paraspinal musculature; costovertebral angle (CVA) tenderness
o Range of motion (flexion, extension, lateral bending, rotation); measure distance from fingertips to floor during forward flexion
o Gait
o Heel/toe walk
o Deep tendon reflexes at knees, ankles (decreased, normal)
o Straight leg raising (SLR)

3 Assessment

o Lumbosacral strain (mild to moderate): Usually patients have reduced range of motion, discomfort that is localized to the lumbosacral area, and palpable muscle tenderness or spasm. Inability to heel/toe walk may be based on increased pain rather than nerve involvement. An SLR that localizes the pain to the lumbosacral area without radiation is considered a negative SLR.
o Nerve root involvement: Disc involvement or sciatica usually is characterized by unilaterally decreased tendon reflexes, foot drop, radiation of pain to the posterior thigh(s), and pain with extension or Valsalva maneuver. Rectal exam may show reduced sphincter tone (*this is a medical emergency*). SLR will be positive for reproducing pain that shoots down the leg.

4 Plan

o Lumbosacral strain usually can be adequately managed by decreasing activity and giving ice massages. Medications, if required, usually consist of anti-inflammatory drugs and/or muscle relaxants.
o Involvement other than mild strains will usually require more extensive management, and a referral is necessary.

5 Medical officer consultation is required in the following cases:

o History of direct trauma to back
o Radiating pain that shoots down the leg
o Marked loss of range of motion
o Severe pain, CVA tenderness, or spinous process tenderness
o Straight leg raise positive
o Bowel or bladder dysfunction

○ Foot drop or unilateral decrease in tendon reflexes
○ When the screener is in doubt or uncomfortable with the case

Minor Trauma

Minor trauma is a very broad topic, the detailed discussion of which is beyond the scope of this manual. Most minor trauma is self-limited, and treatment is largely designed to alleviate pain and protect the patient from further injury. The screener must take caution, however, to rule out more significant injuries, such as fractures, that might be hidden. Blunt trauma to the chest, abdomen, or back, most burns, and significant head injuries always require consultation with or referral to a medical officer. The related discussions on joint pain should be used as cross-reference.

 Subjective

○ Type of trauma (blunt, stretching, compressing, lacerating, penetrating, burn)
○ Location(s) of injury
○ Where, when, and how injury occurred
○ Associated bleeding, loss of consciousness (LOC), nausea and vomiting, dyspnea, weakness, numbness, tingling, loss of mobility
○ Present pain (severity, location, quality, radiation)
○ History of prior trauma to same area
○ Last tetanus shot (date)

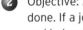 Objective: A complete exam of the injured area(s) should be done. If a joint has been injured, always examine the joint above and below the injured joint.

○ Vital signs
○ Describe size and appearance of wounds
○ Swelling, ecchymosis, deformity
○ Active bleeding
○ Tenderness to palpation, bony point tenderness
○ Pain with voluntary and/or involuntary motion
○ Signs of infection (redness, pus)
○ Distal neurovascular exam (sensation, pulse, capillary refill)

 Assessment

○ Soft tissue injury/contusion: Usually results from blunt or compressing force. Swelling, ecchymosis, and tenderness may be present. No bony point tenderness.

o Superficial laceration: Usually results from sharp trauma. Minimal swelling or tenderness. A laceration is superficial if it does not penetrate below the dermis. An avulsion is an injury in which some of the tissue has been torn away.

o Penetrating wound: Usually results from sharp, penetrating injury. Care must be taken to rule out any foreign body remaining in the wound.

o Abrasion: Superficial scraping or removal of outer layers of skin; minimal bleeding.

o First degree burn: Redness, pain, possibly minimal swelling without blister formation. Almost all sunburns are first degree burns.

o Sprain or strain (grade I): Usually results from stretching or twisting forces across a joint or muscle. There is mild swelling, tenderness, and limitation of motion. See the individual discussions on shoulder, knee, and ankle pain.

o Possible fracture: Fractures may occur with any type of traumatic force. Patients usually have significant swelling, bony point tenderness, and limitation of motion. X-rays are required.

o Do not overlook the fact that a patient may have more than one type of injury at the same time (e.g., contusions, abrasions, and a fracture).

4 Plan

o Soft tissue injuries are treated with cold compresses, rest, and elevation for 24 to 48 hours; use warm compresses to reduce any swelling thereafter. An ace wrap may occasionally be of benefit for pressure and protection. Aspirin, acetaminophen (Tylenol), or ibuprofen (Motrin; consult required) are given to relieve pain.

o Superficial lacerations require thorough irrigation of the wound and cleansing of the surrounding skin using aseptic technique. Gaping lacerations greater than 1 cm in length require referral for possible suturing. Smaller gaping lacerations may be closed with Steri-Strips and dressed.

o Penetrating wounds must be thoroughly irrigated and examined to rule out any foreign body (x-rays may be required). Clean the wound using an angiocatheter connected to normal saline under pressure. Place the catheter into the wound to clean. Do not be timid. If necessary, local anesthetic may be used. *However, be sure the neurologic examination is documented before using a local anesthetic.* Tetanus and antibiotic prophylaxis are sometimes indicated.

o Abrasions must be thoroughly cleansed using aseptic technique and then dressed. Care must be taken to remove all dirt from the wound.

o First degree burns are treated with immediate cold, moist saline ice compresses to decrease pain and cool the skin. The area(s) should then be gently cleansed and rinsed with saline. Dressings are usually not necessary. Emollients may be used to relieve dryness during healing. Aspirin and acetaminophen (Tylenol) often are sufficient analgesics, but codeine may be needed for extensive burns.

- Grade I sprains and strains are treated like soft tissue injuries. The affected joint or muscle should be immobilized with an ace wrap or sling, as appropriate; crutches may be needed for lower extremity injuries. Temporary duty limitations are often indicated.

5 Medical officer consultation is required in the following cases:

- Blunt trauma to abdomen, chest, or back
- History of LOC, nausea, or vomiting
- Facial, hand, and deep or avulsion-type lacerations
- Penetrating wounds to chest or abdomen, or when foreign bodies are possible
- Burns other than first degree or extensive first degree (over 20% of body surface area)
- Significant swelling, ecchymosis
- Bony point tenderness (possible fracture)
- Deformity or severe limitation of motion
- Distal neurovascular abnormality
- Signs of infection present
- Human or animal bites
- When the screener is in doubt or uncomfortable with the case

Nausea and Vomiting

Nausea and vomiting are common, related complaints, and although the most common causes for their occurrence in young adults are mild and self-limited illnesses, there are many serious considerations that must be ruled out. Such a large list is beyond the scope of this manual. The screener must, however, take a thorough history and make referrals as appropriate. The discussions on ABDOMINAL PAIN and HEADACHE should be used as cross-reference.

1 Subjective

- General (onset, frequency, duration, amount vomited)
- Appearance of vomitus (bloody, coffee ground, bilious)
- Associated fever, diarrhea, constipation, abdominal pain, headache, dizziness, or malaise
- Recent appetite

o Jaundice, dark urine, light stools
o Medications, alcohol ingestion
o Dietary range, recent food history
o Pregnancy, last menstrual period (LMP)
o Anxiety, stress

2 Objective

o Vital signs, including postural BP (tilts) and pulse
o Sclera icterus, jaundice; appearance of mucus membranes
o Signs of viral upper respiratory infection (URI) on HEENT exam
o Appearance of abdomen (flat, protuberant, distended)
o Bowel sounds (normal, increased, decreased)
o Tenderness on abdominal palpation
o Guarding or rebound tenderness on palpation
o Guaiac results on any vomitus (if available) or stool

3 Assessment

o Acute gastroenteritis: Nausea and vomiting are frequently accompanied by diarrhea, malaise, and mild fever; occasionally with URI symptoms. Active bowel sounds and little, if any, abdominal tenderness.
o Food poisoning: Similar to gastroenteritis. More often has rapid or sudden onset, with diarrhea following. Clusters of cases with similar food history are seen.
o Following alcohol, drugs: Many chemicals and drugs may cause nausea and vomiting. The exam is usually normal.
o Early pregnancy: LMP greater than 6 weeks ago. Symptoms often worse in morning. Confirm with pregnancy test.
o Migraine headache: Headache is usually the major complaint, but nausea and vomiting may precede a severe headache.
o Acute hepatitis: History similar to gastroenteritis; light stools, dark urine, or jaundice. Right upper quadrant tenderness and liver enlargement are often present.
o Abdominal emergency: Severe abdominal pain, high fever, bloody vomitus or bloody stools.
o Anxiety/stress related: Clear history relating nausea and vomiting to anxiety or stressful event(s). Normal exam.

4 Plan

o Acute gastroenteritis is usually self-limited. Treat with a clear liquid diet, rest, and acetaminophen (Tylenol). If patient cannot hold down fluids, then promethazine (Phenergan) 25 mg IV or per rectum (PR) or prochlorperazine (Compazine) 5 mg IV or PR, may be given (requires consult). Kaopectate or Donnagel may be used for diarrhea.

○ Food poisoning: Same treatment as for gastroenteritis. Report clusters of cases to the preventive medicine team.

○ Following alcohol, drugs: Self-limited, if noxious agent is avoided; withholding the offending medication or referral for special counseling may be required. Dramamine may be of benefit to alleviate symptoms.

○ Early pregnancy: It is best not to give any medications. Symptoms can be minimized by eating several small meals and avoiding high-fat foods.

○ Anxiety/stress related: Reassure patient that no serious organic disease is present. Discuss ways to avoid or alleviate stress; special counseling may be required.

⑤ Medical officer consultation is required in the following cases:

○ Bloody vomitus or coffee-ground appearance
○ Bloody, tarry stools
○ Fever greater than 100°F (37.8°C)
○ Jaundice, icterus
○ Severe headache or dizziness
○ Postural vital signs (BP drops more than 10 mm Hg systolic, pulse rises greater than 20 beats/min, after standing)
○ Abdominal distention
○ Moderate or severe abdominal tenderness
○ Positive guaiac test
○ History of vomiting or persistent vomiting for more than 24 hours
○ When the screener is in doubt or uncomfortable with the case

Nosebleed

The most common sites of nasal bleeding are the mucosal vessels over the cartilaginous nasal septum and the anterior tip of the inferior turbinate. Bleeding is usually caused by external trauma, nose picking, nasal infection from plucking nose hairs, vigorous nose blowing, or drying of the nasal mucosa.

① Subjective

○ Nasal infection
○ Trauma
○ Exposure to drying factors (e.g., sleeping in a closed room with a forced-air heating system)
○ Duration of symptoms

- Pain
- Vigorous nose blowing
- Previous nosebleeds

2 Objective

- Deformity of nose from trauma
- Location of bleeding site
- Vital signs

3 Assessment: Most cases of epistaxis (nosebleed) are uncomplicated. If the problem is recurrent or chronic, other causes must be investigated.

4 Plan

- Most cases can be treated easily by having the patient sit up and lean forward. Tip the head downward and pinch the nose for 5 to 10 minutes. If this does not control the bleeding, then cauterization may be required. A cold pack to the area may also slow the bleeding.
- To prevent recurrence when the cause is dry nasal mucosa, the patient should be given Bacitracin ointment or Nosebetter nasal spray (available over the counter in most drug stores) to use as a protective coating for the nasal mucosa.

5 Medical officer consultation is required for the following cases:

- Significant trauma
- Pain
- BP with systolic greater than 140 mm Hg and diastolic greater than 90 mm Hg
- Pulse greater than 100 beats/min
- Temperature greater than 100°F (37.8°C)
- When pressure does not control bleeding
- Recurrent bleeding episodes
- When the screener is in doubt or uncomfortable with the case

Sexually Transmitted Diseases

Male patients will frequently complain of a burning on urination, a penile discharge, and/or penile lesions. They may describe their problems as clap, drip, or track. Regardless of the slang expression used, medical personnel should approach the problem as being significant and in a serious and professional manner. See CRABS/LICE as a cross-reference.

1 Subjective

o Penile discharge
o Burning on urination (dysuria)
o Fever or chills
o Abdominal or flank pain
o Frequency or urgency of urination
o Genital lesions; description, associated pain
o History of previous sexually transmitted diseases (STDs)

2 Objective

o Vital signs
o Inspect genitals for lesions: describe how they look, location
o Urinalysis if associated with urinary complaints
o Blood sample for VDRL test

3 Assessment

o Gonorrhea usually presents as a thick penile discharge with dysuria, 3 to 7 days after the last sexual contact.
o Nonspecific urethritis usually presents as a thinner penile discharge with dysuria, 4 to 14 days after the last sexual contact.
o Herpes, venereal warts, chancroid, and syphilis all generally present initially with genital lesions.
o Do not overlook the fact that a patient may have more than one type of STD at the same time. In fact, gonorrhea and nonspecific urethritis frequently occur together or with another type of STD.
o Urinary tract infection (UTI): Frequency, urgency, and dysuria accompanied by a low-grade fever suggest an uncomplicated UTI. This is rare in healthy males; however, it should be ruled out by a urinalysis.

4 Plan: Refer to the Epidemiology and Disease Control (EDC) clinic.

5 Medical officer consultation is required in the following cases:

o Female patient
o Genital lesions
o Fever greater than 100°F (37.8°C)
o Abdominal or flank pain
o Patients who return as repeated or questionable treatment failures
o When the screener is in doubt or is uncomfortable with the case

Shoulder Pain

A frequent complaint among active duty soldiers is shoulder pain, usually following strenuous physical activity. The causes of nontraumatic shoulder pain are limited, but there are multiple conditions of traumatic origin, both acute and chronic. Some of the most common causes are listed here.

1 Subjective

- Onset and duration of pain
- Exact location and radiation
- What relieves pain and what makes it worse
- History of activity or trauma
- Prior episodes
- Functional limitations

2 Objective

- Erythema, hot shoulder
- Deformity
- Effusion, pain to palpation (location)
- Active and passive ROM; crepitus
- Strength
- X-ray results, if indicated

3 Assessment

- Rotator cuff tear: Usually presents with shoulder pain/tenderness and a history of trauma. Patient is unable to abduct the arm or hold it abducted against gravity.
- Acute bursitis: Usually produces pain with movement and follows overuse in most instances. Most frequently tender to palpation over subdeltoid bursa.
- Calcific tendonitis: The shoulder may appear swollen and inflamed, and the pain may be severe. X-ray often shows ectopic calcifications.
- Septic arthritis: Should be considered if the patient has a fever or other signs and symptoms of inflammation.
- Dislocation: Usually follows a history of trauma but may occur spontaneously in some people. Sudden onset of pain with gross deformity of shoulder joint and severe limitation of motion. X-ray should be done to rule out associated fracture if there is a history of trauma.
- Referred pain: Shoulder pain may occur with abdominal (subdiaphragmatic) or chest disease or injuries. In these cases the pain is often unrelated to a history of shoulder trauma or to shoulder motion, and there are usually abdominal or chest symptoms.

4 Plan

- Rotator cuff tear is treated initially with a shoulder sling and oral anti-inflammatory drugs (aspirin, Motrin). Many traumatic tears in young patients are significant and may require surgical intervention. Consequently, follow-up with orthopedics is indicated for any patient who does not show significant improvement in pain and increased ROM within 72 hours. Those with improvement should begin a program of ROM and strengthening exercises.

○ Acute bursitis/tendonitis is treated with anti-inflammatory drugs and progressive shoulder exercises. There should be a reduction of certain physical activities, including lifting, push-ups, and pulling, for 7 days.

○ Calcific tendonitis is treated like acute bursitis, but stronger anti-inflammatory drugs may be required for severe pain.

⑤ Medical officer consultation is required in the following cases:

○ Swollen shoulder
○ Hot shoulder/fever
○ Severe pain or deceased ROM
○ Deformity of shoulder (possible dislocation)
○ When the screener is in doubt or uncomfortable with the case

Sinus Complaints

The patient who presents with the complaint of sinusitis may or may not have true sinusitis. Most, in fact, do not. Sinusitis is an infection of the frontal, maxillary, ethmoid, or sphenoid sinuses. The most common pathogens are staphylococci, streptococci, pneumococci, and *Haemophilus influenzae.* Acute sinusitis may follow upper respiratory infection (URI), dental abscess, or nasal allergy.

 Subjective

○ URI complaints
○ Recent dental problems
○ Nasal allergy
○ Headache (location, radiation, relieving and aggravating factors)
○ Facial pain
○ Duration of symptoms
○ Feeling of nasal obstruction
○ Prior history of sinus infection

 Objective

○ Fever
○ Purulent nasal discharge
○ Tenderness to percussion or palpation over frontal and/or maxillary sinuses
○ Injected oropharynx without tonsillar enlargement or exudate

- Appearance of nasal mucosa
- Cough (productive or nonproductive)
- Facial swelling
- Pain when touching chin to chest

3 Assessment

- Boggy, hyperemic nasal mucosa is consistent with allergic rhinitis, the most common cause of sinus complaints. See ALLERGY AND HAY FEVER for discussion.
- Tenderness to percussion over frontal and/or maxillary sinuses is consistent with acute sinusitis.
- Chronic sinusitis may have minimal findings, such as a nasal discharge.

4 Plan

- Allergic rhinitis is best treated by avoidance of the offending allergen. Decongestants and antihistamines are of some benefit.
- Acute or chronic sinusitis will require antibiotics. Analgesics, decongestants, and topical nasal decongestants are also used. A medical officer consultation is required.
- If the ethmoid or sphenoid sinuses are involved, the patient is usually referred to the ear, nose, and throat (ENT) service.

5 Medical officer consultation is required for the following cases:

- Temperature greater than 100°F (37.8°C)
- Retro-orbital headache
- Purulent nasal discharge
- Pain when touching chin to chest
- Tenderness to percussion over maxillary and/or frontal sinuses
- When the screener is in doubt or uncomfortable with the case

Sore Throat

Patients may present with the complaint of sore throat only. The examination should include the following.

1 Subjective

- Duration of symptoms
- Difficulty swallowing or breathing
- Inability to fully open mouth
- Drooling
- Smoking habits

② Objective

- Neck supple
- Elevated temperature
- Oropharynx (injected, edematous)
- Lesions of oral mucosa
- Tonsillar enlargement/exudate
- Cervical adenopathy
- Abdominal tenderness (splenomegaly)

③ Assessment

- *No* significant positive findings: Presumptive viral or irritative pharyngitis (e.g., heavy smoker).
- Injected oropharynx, tonsillar enlargement, exudate: Presumptive beta hemolytic streptococcal (BHS) pharyngitis. Must also have a fever greater than 100°F (37.8°C) with tender cervical adenopathy; rule out mononucleosis if there is also abdominal discomfort.

④ Plan

- Presumptive viral or irritative pharyngitis may be managed by having the patient discontinue smoking and use warm saline or hydrogen peroxide gargles and throat lozenges.
- Presumptive BHS pharyngitis does not need to be confirmed by throat culture if a fever, exudative tonsillitis, and tender cervical adenopathy are present. It may be treated with penicillin, or erythromycin if a penicillin allergy exists. Medical officer consultation or referral is required.
- In certain cases, mononucleosis must also be ruled out. A complete blood count (CBC) with differential is indicated; atypical lymphocytes suggest mononucleosis. A mono spot should also be ordered. A positive reaction is confirmation, but a negative reaction does not exclude mononucleosis.
- Negative mono spots should be repeated in 7 days. The treatment of mononucleosis is basically supportive and may require duty limitations. Antibiotics are not indicated.

⑤ Medical officer consultation is indicated for the following cases:

- Pain when touching chin to chest
- Temperature greater than 100°F (37.8°)
- Difficulty swallowing or breathing
- Inability to fully open mouth or drooling
- Tonsillar enlargement to midline and/or heavy exudate
- When the screener is in doubt or uncomfortable with the case

Superficial Fungal Infections

Multiple forms of superficial fungal infections are found among soldiers. They commonly include infections of the feet, groin, and occasionally the smooth skin (ringworm).

1 Subjective

o Location
o Duration
o Pruritus
o Spread
o Aggravating factors

2 Objective

o Distribution
o Describe lesions (scaly, raised margins, erythematous)
o Superinfection with bacteria from excoriation
o Adenopathy
o Weeping
o Potassium hydroxide (KOH) prep results

3 Assessment: In all cases of suspected fungal infection, a KOH prep is mandatory. A positive KOH is diagnostic; however, a negative KOH does not exclude a fungal infection.

4 Plan

o Fungal infections of the feet, groin, and smooth skin may be treated with clotrimazole (Mycelex or Lotrimin).
o Infections of the nails and hair require oral medication. Topical preparations are ineffective in the treatment of fungal infections of the nails or hair.

5 Medical officer consultation is required in the following cases:

o Significant adenopathy
o Pain
o Involvement of nails or hair
o Infection is deep, rather than superficial
o Lesions appear secondarily infected
o When the screener is in doubt or uncomfortable with the case

Tinea Versicolor

Tinea versicolor is a superficial fungal infection that is most prominent on the upper trunk and arms; it is nonpruritic in most cases. Characterized by hypopigmented, minimally scaling areas, it is more common during hot, humid weather and often recurs from year to year.

1 Subjective

o Onset
o Duration
o Relationship to sun exposure

2 Objective

o Distribution
o Lesions
o KOH prep

3 Assessment: Tinea versicolor is based on hypopigmented, confluent, macular lesions. KOH stain may be positive, with a "spaghetti and meatballs" appearance.

4 Plan: Tinea versicolor is treated with an oral antifungal agent called ketoconazole (Nizoral), which requires a prescription from a medical officer.

5 Medical officer consultation is required for a prescription for the antifungal agent or when the screener is in doubt or uncomfortable with the case.

Upper Respiratory Infection (URI)

Acute infection of the upper airway is characterized by a cough, which may be either productive or nonproductive. Sputum may be mucoid or purulent. There may be a low-grade fever. Rhonchi or wheezing may be heard.

1 Subjective

o Cough (productive or nonproductive)
o Feeling of stuffiness in ears
o Stiff neck
o Hoarseness
o Sore throat

o Runny nose
o Increased lacrimation
o Chest pain during cough or during inspiration
o Duration of symptoms

2 Objective

o Neck (supple, presence of pain when touching chin to chest)
o Eyes (conjunctival injection, photophobia)
o Tympanic membranes (appearance)
o Nasal discharge (mucoid, purulent)
o Oropharynx (injected, tonsillar enlargement, exudates)
o Cervical adenopathy
o Chest (rhonchi, wheezing)

3 Assessment: Based on examination.

4 Plan: Most uncomplicated URIs can be managed with antihistamines, decongestants, antitussives for moderate to severe cough, and aspirin or acetaminophen for elevated temperature or sore throat.

5 Medical officer consultation is indicated in the following cases:

o Temperature greater than 100°F (37.8°C)
o Pain when touching chin to chest
o Purulent sputum, dark sputum
o Hoarseness for 1 week
o Eardrum bulging
o Tonsils grossly swollen, necrotic, or heavily exudative
o Difficulty in swallowing
o Symptoms present for more than 1 week
o If the screener is in doubt or uncomfortable with the case

Guidelines for Seeking Medical Officer Consultation During Patient Triage

Patients with the following signs and symptoms should be brought to the attention of a medical officer immediately. These guidelines will serve you well in the battalion aid station (BAS), temporary mobilization center (TMC), or in the emergency room of a U.S. Army Medical Center (MEDCEN). Of course, if you ever feel uncomfortable with any patient, obtain medical officer consultation.

Bleeding

- Suspected posterior epistaxis (bleeding in the back of the nose)
- Epistaxis uncontrolled by 10 minutes of medically supervised nasal pressure (i.e., bleeding does not stop during appropriately applied nasal pressure)
- Hematochezia (bloody stools), melena (dark, tarry stools), or history of same
- Hematemesis (vomiting blood)
- Anticoagulated patients with bleeding
- For vaginal bleeding, see OBSTETRIC AND GYNECOLOGIC PROBLEMS

Blood Pressure: Increased (diastolic greater than 110 mm Hg)

- See VITAL SIGNS

Chest Pain

- New or changing angina (definition: spasmodic, choking, suffocating chest pain)
- Suspicion of unstable angina or myocardial infarction (change in anginal pattern)
- Chest pain associated with heart rate over 100 or less than 50 or with an irregular pulse
- Chest pain associated with systolic blood pressure less than 90 mm Hg or diastolic greater than 115 mm Hg
- Chest pain with dyspnea
- Chest pain associated with new ECG findings
- Chest pain associated with systolic blood pressure difference of more than 20 mm Hg between left and right arms or a history suspicious for aortic dissection
- Chest pain in a drug abuser

Eye Complaints

- Abrupt loss or significant decrease of vision (greater than one-line change in visual acuity)
- Associated amaurosis fugax (transient loss of vision in one eye), burst of floaters, abrupt flashes of light, halos, or waving curtains
- Eye trauma or foreign body embedded in cornea
- Eye pain around globe or socket (not irritation)
- Chemical injury (battery acid, etc.)

o Diplopia (new onset in less than 48 hours)
o Facial herpes or varicella zoster with eye or nose tip involvement
o High-speed foreign body injury (from lawnmower, table saw, etc.)

Fever

o Adult
  ■ In any suspected IV drug abuser
  ■ Associated with threat to airway
  ■ Associated with meningeal signs
  ■ Associated with altered mental status
o Children (older than 24 months) who appear toxic at any temperature or with temperature greater than 104°F (40°C)
o Toddler or infants (between 3 months to 24 months) with a temperature (rectal) greater than or equal to 103°F (39.5°C) or if the patient appears toxic at any temperature
o Neonates (less than 12 weeks) with rectal temperatures greater than 100.4°F (38°C) or less than 96.5°F (35.8°C)

Headaches

o With meningeal signs or suspected meningitis
o With persistent vomiting, fever, photophobia, neck pain with movement
o With associated neurologic alteration
o Associated with recent trauma
o In patients who relate abrupt onset of the most intense headache they've ever had or in patients with history of migraine headaches who have new type of severe headache
o Associated with diastolic blood pressure greater than 110 mm Hg
o Associated with significant vision disturbances (decreased visual acuity greater than one line from other eye or prior exam)
o Associated with syncope

Infection

o Abscesses with fever or malaise/weakness, especially in immuno-compromised patient (HIV, cancer, diabetes, on steroids, splenectomized, etc.)
o Perirectal abscess
o Pilonidal cyst

Insect, Spider, or Snake Bites or Allergic Reactions

o Within 4 hours
o Swelling above next major joint on extremity wounds

- Shortness of breath or wheezing
- Chest tightness
- Sense of swelling in throat
- Associated with generalized rash
- Intense pain, as with black widow spider bites
- History of allergic response to similar bite or sting
- Petechiae
- Suspected *Loxosceles* envenomation (bite from brown recluse spider)
- All snakebites

Neurologic

- Suspected current or recent transient ischemic attack (TIA) or stroke
- Altered mental status
- Any paralysis

Obstetric and Gynecologic Problems

- Crowning (definition: large segment of the fetal scalp visible within the vagina)
- Imminent delivery
- Suspected ectopic pregnancy (pain, vaginal bleeding, and known pregnancy)
- Nonpregnant vaginal hemorrhage associated with positive tilts or tachycardia at rest
- Vaginal bleeding in pregnancy of less than 20 weeks
- Vaginal bleeding in pregnancy of more than 20 weeks
- Alleged rape or sexual assault
- Pregnancy with blood pressure greater than 140/90 mm Hg or a 20 mm Hg rise from patient's baseline, or proteinuria with headache or abdominal pain (think of toxemia of pregnancy)

Overdose or Poison Ingestion

- Anyone with suspected poison ingestion or overdose

Pain

- Abdominal pain associated with mass, especially if it is pulsatile
- Intractable, severe abdominal pain
- Eye pain (not irritation)
- Suspected deep vein thrombosis

Pediatrics

- Fever: See FEVER
- Head injury in a 2-year-old or younger, or any age with neurologic deficits
- Any child who appears toxic or lethargic
- Any child with recent viral illness and a single episode of vomiting who behaves unusually
- Cyanosis
- Child younger than 5 years who is unable to use an extremity
- Suspected Child Abuse and/or Neglect (SCAN)
- Vomiting in first 8 weeks of life (not regurgitating)
- Children with respiratory distress or wheezing

Psychiatric Problems

- Patients who pose a threat to themselves or others
- Psychotic or delusional patients
- All paranoid schizophrenics with active symptoms
- Alcohol detoxification requests

Respiratory Complaints

- Shortness of breath with respiratory rate greater than 24 breaths/min in an adult
- Respiratory distress (tachypnea with respiratory distress)
- Shortness of breath associated with systolic blood pressure less than 90 mm Hg or diastolic greater than 115 mm Hg
- Shortness of breath associated with pulse less than 50 or greater than 120
- Dyspnea associated with foreign body ingestion or aspiration
- History of choking on a foreign body
- Dyspnea with cyanosis
- Dyspnea with risk factors suggestive of pulmonary embolism: tachypnea, tachycardia, ECG changes, or any chest pains
- Tachypnea associated with chemstrip showing blood sugar level greater than 240
- Exacerbation of asthma or chronic obstructive pulmonary disease (COPD) by history: respiratory distress with or without wheezing
- Urticaria with wheezing or oral/facial swelling

Seizures

- Actively seizing
- Seizure within 2 hours
- New-onset seizure
- Change in normal seizure pattern
- Altered mental status

Syncope

- In all patients without obvious vasovagal cause (e.g., needlestick)
- With associated trauma (either before or after)
- Secondary to heat injury
- With positive tilts or symptoms

Trauma

- Lacerations less than 24 hours old or facial lacerations of any duration that may result in significant disfigurement
- Trauma less than 24 hours old
- Closed head trauma with neurologic changes or in a child under 2 years of age
- Trauma with associated chest pain or shortness of breath
- Trauma less than 24 hours old with associated hematuria
- Assault within 24 hours (except sexual assault—consult every time)
- All animal or human bites (for insect bites see INSECT, SPIDER, OR SNAKE BITES OR ALLERGIC REACTIONS)
- Closed adult extremity injuries, less than 24 hours old, with accompanying x-rays (where indicated)
- Pediatric (younger than 12 years old) extremity injuries, less than 48 hours old, with accompanying x-rays (where indicated)
- From a major mechanism of injury (motor vehicle accident, low-altitude entanglement, etc.)

Urinary Complaints

- Unable to pass any urine
- Suspected renal stone (pain and hematuria)
- Patients with a toxic appearance who have urinary tract infections
- Patients older than 55 or with complex medical histories, with temperature over 101°F (38.2°C) with pyuria

Vital Signs

> **note**
>
> The medic should personally recheck abnormal vital signs manually.

- Adult
    - Heart rate < 50 or > 120 beats/min resting
    - BP systolic < 90 mm Hg or diastolic > 115 mm Hg
    - Respiratory rate > 24 or < 10 breaths/min
- Pediatric
    - Younger than 5 years: Heart rate > 180 or < 80 beats/min
    - Older than 5 years: Heart rate > 160 or < 60 beats/min, or respiratory rate > 60 breaths/min

Vomiting

- Associated loss of consciousness
- Hematemesis
- Associated head injury
- Systolic blood pressure less than 90 mm Hg
- Associated visual complaints
- Acute or surgical abdomen
- Orthostatic signs and/or symptoms
- Associated orthostatic pulse increase of greater than 20 beats/min or systolic blood pressure drop greater than 10 mm Hg with orthostatic symptoms
- Suspected drug toxicity
- Cancer patients
- Associated altered mental status

Fractures and Splinting

A fracture is any break in the continuity of a bone. Fractures can cause total disability or in some cases death. On the other hand, they can most often be treated so that there is complete recovery. A great deal depends upon the first aid the individual receives before he or she is moved. First aid includes immobilizing the fractured part in addition to applying lifesaving measures. The basic splinting principle is to immobilize the joints above and below any fracture.

Figure 10 Closed fracture.

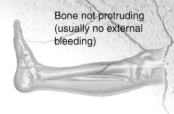

Bone not protruding
(usually no external
bleeding)

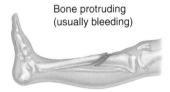

Bone protruding
(usually bleeding)

Open fracture

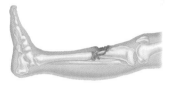

Open fracture
produced by missile

Figure 11 Open fractures.

Kinds of Fractures

- ○ Closed fracture: A broken bone that does not break the overlying skin (**Figure 10**). Tissue beneath the skin may be damaged.
- ○ Dislocation: A joint, such as a knee, ankle, or shoulder, that is not in proper position. Dislocations should be treated as closed fractures.
- ○ Sprain: Occurs when the connecting tissues of the joints have been torn. Sprains should be treated as closed fractures.
- ○ Open fracture: A broken bone that breaks (pierces) the overlying skin (**Figure 11**). The broken bone may come through the skin, or a missile such as a bullet or shell fragment may go through the flesh and break the bone. An open fracture is contaminated and subject to infection.

Signs and Symptoms of Fractures

Indications of a fracture are deformity, tenderness, swelling, and pain; an inability to move the injured part; and protruding bone, bleeding, or discolored skin at the injury site. A sharp pain when the individual attempts to move the part is also a sign of a fracture. *Do not* encourage the casualty to move the injured part in order to identify a fracture, since such movement could cause further damage to surrounding tissues and promote shock. If you are not sure whether a bone is fractured, treat the injury as a fracture.

Purposes of Immobilizing Fractures

A fracture is immobilized to prevent the sharp edges of the bone from moving and cutting tissue, muscle, blood vessels, and nerves. This reduces pain and helps prevent or control shock. In a closed fracture, immobilization keeps bone fragments from causing an open wound and prevents contamination and possible infection. Splint to immobilize.

Splints, Padding, Bandages, Slings, and Swathes

○ Splints: May be improvised from such items as boards, poles, sticks, tree limbs, rolled magazines, rolled newspapers, or cardboard. If nothing is available for a splint, the chest wall can be used to immobilize a fractured arm, and the uninjured leg can be used to immobilize (to some extent) the fractured leg.

○ Padding: May be improvised from such items as a jacket, blanket, poncho, shelter half, or leafy vegetation.

○ Bandages: May be improvised from belts, rifle slings, bandoliers, kerchiefs, or strips torn from clothing or blankets. Narrow materials such as wire or cord should not be used to secure a splint in place.

○ Slings: A sling is a bandage (or improvised material such as a piece of cloth, a belt, and so forth) suspended from the neck to support an upper extremity. Slings may also be improvised by using the tail of a coat or shirt or using pieces torn from such items as clothing and blankets. The triangular bandage is ideal for this purpose. Remember that the casualty's hand should be higher than his or her elbow, and the sling should be applied so that the supporting pressure is on the uninjured side.

○ Swathes: Any bands (pieces of cloth, pistol belts, and so forth) that are used to further immobilize a splinted fracture. Triangular and cravat bandages are often used as or referred to as swathe bandages. The purpose of the swathe is to immobilize; therefore, the swathe bandage is placed above and/or below the fracture—not over it.

Splinting Suspected Fractures

Before beginning first aid treatment for a fracture, gather whatever splinting materials are available. Materials may consist of splints, such as wooden boards, branches, or poles. Other splinting materials include padding, improvised cravats, and/or bandages. Ensure that splints are long enough to immobilize the joint above and below the suspected fracture. If possible, use at least four ties (two above and two below the fracture) to secure the splints. The ties should be non-slip knots and should be tied away from the body on the splint.

Performance Steps

1 Evaluate the casualty.

○ Be prepared to perform any necessary lifesaving measures. Monitor the casualty for development of conditions that may require you to perform necessary basic lifesaving measures. These measures include clearing the airway, performing rescue breathing, preventing shock, and/or controlling bleeding.

▼ WARNING

Unless there is immediate life-threatening danger, such as a fire or an explosion, *do not* move the casualty with a suspected back or neck injury. Improper movement may cause permanent paralysis or death.

▼ WARNING

In a chemical environment, *do not* remove any of the casualty's protective clothing. Apply the dressing/splint over the clothing.

2 Locate the site of the suspected fracture.

○ Ask the casualty for the location of the injury. Is there any pain? Where is it tender? Can he or she move the extremity?
○ Look for an unnatural position of the extremity. Look for a bone sticking out (protruding).

3 Prepare the casualty for splinting the suspected fracture.

○ Reassure the casualty. Tell the casualty that you will be taking care of him or her and that medical aid is on the way.
○ Loosen any tight or binding clothing.
○ Remove all the jewelry from the casualty and place it in the casualty's pocket. Tell the casualty you are doing this because if the jewelry is not removed at this time and swelling occurs later, further bodily injury can occur.

> **note** ──────────────────────────────────
>
> Boots should not be removed from the casualty unless they are needed to stabilize a neck injury or there is actual bleeding from the foot.

4 Gather splinting materials.

- If standard splinting materials (splints, padding, cravats, and so forth) are not available, gather improvised materials. Splints can be improvised from wooden boards, tree branches, poles, or rolled newspapers or magazines.
- Splints should be long enough to reach beyond the joints above and below the suspected fracture site.
- Improvised padding, such as a jacket, blanket, poncho, shelter half, or leafy vegetation may be used. A cravat can be improvised from a piece of cloth, a large bandage, a shirt, or a towel.
- To immobilize a suspected fracture of an arm or a leg, parts of the casualty's body may also be used. For example, the chest wall may be used to immobilize an arm, and the uninjured leg may be used to immobilize the injured leg.

> **note** ──────────────────────────────────
>
> If splinting material is not available and the suspected fracture *cannot* be splinted, then swathes or a combination of swathes and slings can be used to immobilize an extremity.

5 Pad the splints.

- Pad the splints where they touch any bony part of the body, such as the elbow, wrist, knee, ankle, crotch, or armpit. Padding prevents excessive pressure to the area.

6 Check the circulation below the site of the injury.

- Note any pale, white, or bluish-gray color of the skin, which may indicate impaired circulation. Circulation can also be checked by depressing the toe or finger nailbeds and observing how quickly the color returns. A slower return of pink color to the injured side when compared with the uninjured side indicates a problem with circulation. Depressing the toe or finger nailbeds is the method to use to check the circulation in a dark-skinned casualty.

- Check the temperature of the injured extremity. Use your hand to compare the temperature of the injured side with the uninjured side of the body. The body area below the injury may be colder to the touch, indicating poor circulation.
- Question the casualty about the presence of numbness, tightness, cold, or tingling sensations.

▼ WARNING

Casualties with fractures to the extremities may show impaired circulation, such as numbness, tingling, cold, and/or pale to blue skin. These casualties should be evacuated by medical personnel and treated as soon as possible. Prompt medical treatment may prevent possible loss of the limb.

▼ WARNING

If it is an open fracture (i.e., skin is broken; bone(s) may be sticking out), *do not attempt to push bone(s) back under the skin*. Apply a field dressing to protect the area.

7 Apply the splint in place.

- Splint the fracture(s) in the position found. *Do not* attempt to reposition or straighten the injury. If it is an open fracture, stop the bleeding and protect the wound. Cover all wounds with field dressings before applying a splint. Remember to use the casualty's field dressing, not your own. If bones are protruding (sticking out), *do not* attempt to push them back under the skin. Apply dressings to protect the area.
- Place one splint on each side of the arm or leg. If possible, the splints should reach beyond the joints above and below the fracture.
- Tie the splints. Secure each splint in place above and below the fracture site with improvised (or actual) cravats. Improvised cravats can be made from such things as strips of cloth, belts, or whatever else you have. With minimal motion to the injured areas, place and tie the splints with the bandages. Push cravats through and under the natural body curvatures (spaces), and then gently position the improvised cravats and tie in place. Use nonslip knots. Tie all knots on the splint away from the casualty (**Figure 12**). *Do not* tie cravats directly over a suspected fracture or dislocation site.

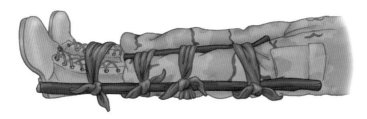

Figure 12   Nonslip knots tied away from casualty.

8   Check the splint for tightness.

o Check to be sure that bandages are tight enough to securely hold the splinting materials in place, but not so tight that circulation is impaired.

o Recheck the circulation after application of the splint. Check the skin color and temperature. This is to ensure that the bandages holding the splint in place have not been tied too tightly. A fingertip check can be made by inserting the tip of the finger between the wrapped tails and the skin.

o Make any adjustment necessary without allowing the splint to become ineffective.

9   Apply a sling if applicable.

o An improvised sling may be made from any available nonstretching piece of cloth, such as a fatigue shirt or trouser, poncho, or shelter half. Slings may also be improvised using the tail of a coat, a belt, or a piece of cloth from a blanket or some clothing. See **Figure 13** for a shirt tail used for support. A pistol belt or trouser belt also may be used for support (**Figure 14**).

o A sling should place the supporting pressure on the casualty's uninjured side. The supported arm should have the hand positioned slightly higher than the elbow.

Upper Extremity Fractures

Figure 15 shows how to apply slings, splints, and cravats (swathes) to immobilize and support fractures of the upper extremities. Although the padding is not visible in some of the illustrations, it is always preferable to apply padding along the injured part for the length of the splint, especially where the splint touches any bony parts of the body.

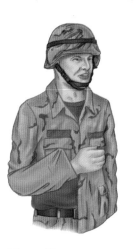

Figure 13 Shirt tail used for support.

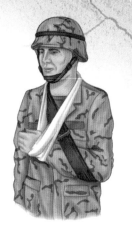

Figure 14 Belt used for support.

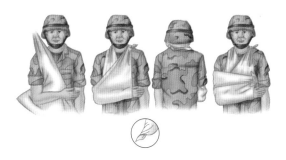

A

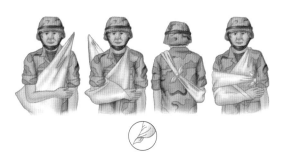

B

Figure 15 Application of triangular bandage to form a sling. A: Method 1.
B: Method 2.

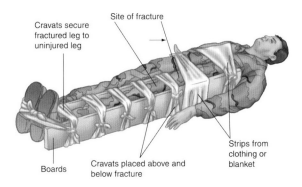

Cravats secure
fractured leg to
uninjured leg

Site of fracture

Boards

Cravats placed above and
below fracture

Strips from
clothing or
blanket

Figure 16   Board splint applied to fractured hip or thigh.

Lower Extremity Fractures

Figure 16 shows how to apply slings, splints, and cravats (swathes) to immobilize and support fractures of the lower extremities. Padding should be applied along the injured part for the length of the splint, especially where the splint touches any bony parts of the body.

Shock Management
Causes and Effects

o Shock may be caused by severe or minor trauma to the body. It usually is the result of the following:
   ▪ Significant loss of blood
   ▪ Heart failure
   ▪ Dehydration
   ▪ Severe and painful blows to the body
   ▪ Severe burns of the body
   ▪ Severe wound infections
   ▪ Severe allergic reactions to drugs, foods, insect stings, and snakebites
o Shock stuns and weakens the body. When the normal blood flow in the body is upset, death can result. Early identification and proper treatment may save the casualty's life.
o See FM 8-230 for further information and details on specific types of shock and treatment.

Signs and Symptoms

○ Examine the casualty to see if he or she has any of the following signs or symptoms.

- Sweaty but cool skin (clammy skin)
- Paleness of skin
- Restlessness, nervousness
- Thirst
- Loss of blood (bleeding)
- Confusion (or loss of awareness)
- Faster-than-normal breathing rate
- Blotchy or bluish skin (especially around the mouth and lips)
- Nausea and/or vomiting

Treatment and Prevention

In the field, the procedures to treat shock are identical to procedures that would be performed to prevent shock. When treating a casualty, assume that shock is present or will occur shortly. By waiting until actual signs or symptoms of shock are noticeable, the rescuer may jeopardize the casualty's life.

Performance Steps

1 Position the casualty. (*Do not* move the casualty or the casualty's limbs if suspected fractures have not been splinted.)

2 Move the casualty to cover, if cover is available and the situation permits.

3 Lay the casualty on his or her back.

> **note**
>
> A casualty in shock after suffering a heart attack, chest wound, or breathing difficulty may breathe easier in a sitting position. If this is the case, allow the casualty to sit upright, but monitor carefully in case his or her condition worsens.

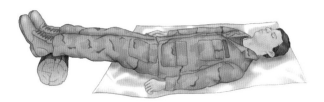

Figure 17   Casualty with clothing loosened and feet elevated.

4   Elevate the casualty's feet higher than the level of his or her heart (**Figure 17**).

o Use a stable object (a box, field pack, or rolled-up clothing) so that the casualty's feet will not slip.

▼ WARNING

Do not elevate legs if the casualty has an unsplinted broken leg, head injury, or abdominal injury.

▼ WARNING

Check casualty for leg fracture(s) and splint, if necessary, before elevating the feet. For a casualty with an abdominal wound, place knees in an upright (flexed) position.

5   Loosen clothing at the neck, waist, or wherever it may be binding (see **Figure 17**).

CAUTION

Do not loosen or remove protective clothing in a chemical environment.

6   Prevent chilling or overheating.

o The key is to maintain body temperature (**Figure 18**).

o In cold weather, and in all trauma patients, place a blanket or other like item over the casualty to keep him or her warm and under the

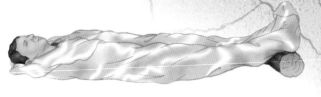

Figure 18 Body temperature maintained.

casualty to prevent chilling. However, if a tourniquet has been applied, leave it exposed (if possible).

○ In hot weather, place the casualty in the shade and avoid excessive covering.

7 Calm the casualty.

○ Throughout the entire procedure of treating and caring for a casualty, the rescuer should reassure the casualty and keep him or her calm. This can be done by being authoritative (taking charge) and by showing self-confidence. Assure the casualty that you are there to help him or her.

> ⚠**WARNING**
>
> During the treatment and prevention of shock, *do not* give the casualty any food or drink. If you must leave the casualty or if the casualty is unconscious, turn his or her head to the side to prevent the casualty from choking should he or she vomit.

8 Seek medical aid.

9 Evaluate casualty: If necessary, continue with the casualty's evaluation.

Administering Blood

Performance Steps

1 Verify and inspect the blood pack received from the laboratory.

○ Note the time the blood pack was received and record the time on the SF 518 form.

note

Infusion of a blood pack should be initiated within
30 minutes of being issued.

○ Two people must verify and match the information on the blood
pack label with the data on the requisition form (SF 518).

note

One of the verifiers must be a registered nurse when
directed by local policy.

○ Inspect the blood for abnormalities such as gas bubbles or black or
gray-colored sediment (indicative of bacterial growth).

note

Return the blood pack to the blood bank if any abnormality is present or suspected.

○ Match the blood pack with the patient's identification.
  ■ The same two people must compare the information on the blood
  unit with the data on the patient's wristband. Ensure that the
  patient's name, blood type, and hospital number positively match
  the data on the blood pack.
  ■ Sign the SF 518 in accordance with local policy when all the data
  has been confirmed as a positive match.

2 Establish baseline data.

○ Reconfirm data from the patient's history regarding allergies or pre-
vious reactions to blood or blood products.
○ Measure and evaluate the vital signs.
○ Record the vital signs on the SF 518 and in the nursing notes.

3 Prepare the blood and the blood recipient set.

note

Use only tubing that is designed for the administration
of blood products. It is equipped with a filter designed
for the fine filtration required for blood products.

- Close all three clamps on the Y tubing.
- Aseptically insert one of the tubing spikes into the container of normal saline. Invert and hang this container about 3 feet above the level of the patient.
- Open the clamp on the normal saline line and prime the upper line and the blood filter.
- Open the clamp on the empty line on which you will eventually hang the blood. Normal saline will flow up the empty line to prime that portion of the tubing.

> **note**
>
> Use only 0.9% normal saline for injection with blood. Other solutions are not compatible.

- Once the blood line is primed with saline, close the clamp on the blood line.
- Leave the clamp on the normal saline line open.
- Open the main roller clamp to prime the lower infusion tubing.
- Close the main roller clamp.
- Aseptically expose the blood port on the blood pack.
- Aseptically insert the remaining spike into the blood port and hang the blood at the same level as the normal saline container.

> **note**
>
> If Y-type recipient tubing is not available, use regular infusion tubing for the normal saline and the available blood recipient tubing for the blood pack. Prime each set. Attach a sterile, large-bore (16- or 18-gauge) needle to the end of the blood tubing and "piggyback" the blood into the normal saline line below the level of the roller clamp. Hang the blood pack at least 6 inches higher than the normal saline.

4 Perform the venipuncture.

> **note**
>
> Insert a large-gauge (14, 16, or 18) IV catheter for administering blood to an adult patient. This will enhance the flow of blood and prevent hemolysis of the cells.

5 Begin the infusion of blood.

o Attach the primed infusion set to the catheter, tape it securely, and open the main roller clamp.

note

If a pre-existing catheter is being used, run in 50 cc of normal saline to flush out any incompatible solution. If a new catheter was inserted, this step is not required.

o Close the roller clamp to the normal saline and open the roller clamp to the blood.

o Adjust the flow rate with the main roller clamp.

■ Set the flow rate to deliver approximately 10 to 25 cc of blood over the first 15 minutes.

note

When delivering blood by piggyback, begin the infusion by opening the roller clamp on the normal saline line and setting it to a TKO (to keep open) rate. Adjust the roller clamp on the blood line to deliver 10 to 25 cc of blood over the first 15 minutes.

■ Monitor the vital signs closely for the first 15 minutes and observe for indications of an adverse reaction to the blood.

CAUTION

Any time an adverse reaction is suspected, immediately stop the blood and infuse normal saline. Notify the charge nurse and physician immediately.

■ Set the main roller clamp to deliver the prescribed flow rate if, after the first 15 minutes, no adverse reaction is suspected and the vital signs are stable.

note

Use the correct formula to calculate flow rate.

6   Monitor and evaluate the patient throughout the procedure.

- Monitor vital signs every hour or more frequently in accordance with local standard operating procedure (SOP).
- Compare the vital signs with previous and baseline vital signs.
- Observe for changes that indicate an adverse reaction to the blood.
- Stop the blood, infuse normal saline, and notify the charge nurse and physician if a reaction is suspected.

> **CAUTION**
>
> When a transfusion reaction occurs or is suspected, the unused blood and recipient tubing must be sent to the laboratory along with a 10-mL specimen of the patient's venous blood and a post-transfusion urine specimen.

7   Discontinue the infusion of blood.

- When the blood pack has emptied, close the clamp to the blood and open the clamp to the normal saline.
- Flush the tubing and filter with approximately 50 cc of normal saline to deliver the residual blood.
- After the residual blood has been delivered, run the normal saline at a TKO rate or hang another solution, if one has been prescribed.
- Take and record the vital signs at the completion of the transfusion and 1 hour after completion.

> **note**
>
> As a rule, a unit of blood should be infused within 2 to 4 hours unless contraindicated by risk of circulatory overload. If the prescribed flow rate will deliver the blood within a shorter or longer period of time, verify the order with the charge nurse or prescribing physician.

8   Dispose of the used blood pack in accordance with local SOP.

- Return it to the laboratory blood bank with a copy of SF 518.
- Discard it in a container for contaminated waste.

9   Document the procedure and significant nursing observations on the appropriate forms in accordance with local SOP.

o Complete the SF 518.
- Return one copy to the laboratory blood bank.
- Place one copy in the patient's chart.
o Record the procedure and the patient's response in a nursing note entry.

Administering Blood Products

Performance Steps

1 Verify the privileged provider's order and ensure that the patient has a current signed informed consent for transfusion.

2 Review the procedure for administering a blood transfusion.

CAUTION

The administration of blood and blood products is generally outside the scope of practice of the 91WM6. Administration of blood and blood products is restricted to the domain of a privileged provider or registered nurse. However, this task is an expected skill of the 91WM6 in a combat field environment.

3 Obtain the blood component from the blood bank.

4 Obtain the appropriate administration set.

5 Review the directions and facility protocol for administration of the blood product.

o Rate of administration
o Route
o Risk factors
o Possible complications

6 Obtain a positive identification of the patient and provide privacy.

7 Wash your hands and follow standard precautions.

8 Explain the procedure to the patient and/or family.

9 Administer the prescribed blood product.

> **note**
>
> When using an infusion control device (pump), review the manufacturer's instructions for use to ensure you are using the correct pump, configured correctly, with the proper tubing and filter.

- Fresh plasma: Rapid administration with straight-line administration set.
- Platelets: Administer at a rate of 10 minutes per unit, using the platelet infusion set and filter.
- Granulocytes: Slow administration over 2 to 4 hours with Y-type blood tubing and normal saline. Do not use a microaggregate filter.
- Serum albumin: Slow administration at 1 mL/min using the special tubing supplied with the solution.
- Gamma globulin: Given IM 0.25 to 0.5 mL.
- Coagulation factors: Administer with standard syringe or component drip set.
  - Factor VIII: 1 unit per 5 minutes
  - Factor IX: Reconstitute 10 to 20 mL of diluent

10 Monitor the patient for unexpected outcomes and report abnormal findings to the charge nurse or privileged provider.

11 Conduct patient education based on specific patient needs.

12 Document the nursing activity.

- Type and amount of blood product administered
- Volume of saline or diluent used
- Patient's response to the procedure
- Unexpected outcomes and interventions
- Patient education provided

Calculating an IV Flow Rate

- Information required to determine flow rate:
  - Total volume to be infused.
  - Time period over which it is to be infused.
  - Properties of the administration set (how many drops per milliliter it delivers); this information is found on the box containing the administration set.

○ Formula for calculating IV flow rate:

$$\frac{\text{Volume to be infused} \times \text{Drops/mL of infusion set}}{\text{Total time of infusion in minutes}}$$

Examples

○ SFC Murray received a physician's order to administer an intravenous infusion. The order states that the total volume of 1,000 mL is to be delivered over a 4-hour period. The IV set that is to be used will deliver 20 drops per milliliter. How many drops per minute (gtt/min) should be administered?

  1. Total volume to be infused = 1,000 mL

  2. Infusion set (drops/mL) = 20

  3. Total time of infusion = 240 min (4 hr × 60 min)

  4. Multiply 1,000 × 20 = 20,000; then divide by 240 = 83.33

$$\frac{1000 \times 20}{240 \text{ min}} = \frac{20,000}{240} = 83.33$$

  5. Drops per minute = 83.33; round to 83 gtt/min

○ CPT Smith's IV is ordered at 150 mL, to be delivered over 1 hour. The administration set being used delivers 20 gtt/mL. Calculate the drops per minute to be administered.

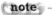

note

Use the same formula as the previous example.

  1. Total volume to be infused = 150 mL

  2. Infusion set (drops/mL) = 20

  3. Total time of infusion = 60 min

  4. Multiply 150 × 20 = 3,000; then divide by 60 = 50 gtt/min

$$\frac{150 \times 20}{60} = \frac{3000}{60} = 50$$

Summary

Shock is a state of inadequate tissue perfusion that can be caused by a variety of disease states and injuries. If the syndrome is severe or prolonged, it may become irreversible, resulting in multiple organ failure and death. Initiating and maintaining an IV infusion may make a difference between saving or losing a patient's life. The ability to properly calculate and regulate the flow of IV fluid is essential to the care of the patient with an IV.

Administering Intravenous and Intramuscular Medications

Purpose, Needle Characteristics, and Sites for Intramuscular (IM) Injections

- Purpose
  - Used when rapid absorption or rate of onset (10 to 20 minutes) and long duration (hours to weeks) are desired.
  - Used when administering viscous or irritating medications.
  - Used when a large volume of medication is needed for a stronger effect.

    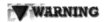 **WARNING**

    Because absorption of medications administered by the intramuscular route relies on adequate blood flow to the muscles, IM injections should not be used in individuals with poor circulation or symptoms of shock.

- Needle characteristics
  - Not less than 1 inch for an adult. You may use a smaller size if the patient is thin.
  - May need up to a 2-inch needle for obese patients.

    CAUTION

    Selection of a needle long enough to reach the muscle is essential. Using a needle that is too short will cause the medication to be injected into subcutaneous tissue, potentially reducing absorption and effectiveness.

  - Gauge (diameter) range: 20 to 22
- Primary IM injection sites
  - Deltoid muscle
    - Used for medication volumes up to 2 mL in an adult.
    - Faster absorption than other IM sites.

- Muscle is located in the outer one third of the arm between the shoulder bone (acromion process) and axilla.
  - Injection site is approximately three finger-widths below the shoulder bone, in the middle of the deltoid muscle mass.
- Gluteus maximus
  - Used for larger medication volumes, up to 5 mL.
  - May require a long needle (2 inches or longer in large adults).
  - Located by dividing one buttock into four imaginary quadrants—injection area is in upper, outer quadrant.

CAUTION

An injection given in an area outside this site could cause damage to the sciatic nerve or puncture the superior gluteal artery, causing either paralysis or severe bleeding. *Use extreme care when identifying the gluteal site!*

- Vastus lateralis
  - One of the safest sites due to the absence of major nerves and blood vessels.
  - May be more painful due to the number of small nerve endings.
  - Medication volume up to 5 mL in adults.
  - Muscle mass is on lateral thigh.
  - Injection site extends from the middle of the anterior thigh to the middle of the lateral thigh, and from one hand's width below the hip joint to one hand's width above the knee.
○ Length and gauge selected will vary depending on the amount of muscle mass and the age, size, and condition of the patient.

Purpose, Needle Characteristics, and Sites for Subcutaneous (SQ) Injections

○ Purpose
  - Used when absorption rate desired is slower than that provided by the IM route. The absorption rate for SQ injection is 15 to 30 minutes. Duration is comparable to IM route: hours to weeks.
  - Used for small amounts of watery and nonirritating medications.
○ Needle characteristics
  - Length: 0.5 inch to 1 inch.
  - Gauge (diameter) range: 23 to 25.
  - Selection of needle length and gauge will vary depending on the amount of subcutaneous tissue and the age, size, and condition of the patient.

- Sites
  - Upper arm
    - Rear lateral aspect.
    - Injection area is approximately one hand's width down from the shoulder and one third of the way around laterally.
    - Medication volume: Not to exceed 0.5 mL.
  - Vastus lateralis
    - Injection site extends from the middle of the anterior thigh to the middle of the lateral thigh, and from one hand's width below the hip joint to one hand's width above the knee.
    - Medication volume: Not to exceed 2 mL.
  - Abdomen
    - Medications such as insulin and heparin are administered in the subcutaneous tissue of the abdomen.
    - The amount of medication given will vary according to the needs of the patient.
    - A physician will prescribe the dosage to be given in the abdomen.

Preparation and Administration of Intramuscular and Subcutaneous Injections

Performance Steps for Preparation

1 Identify the patient.

2 Verify the required injection(s).
- Check the physician's order.
- Review the patient's medical record to identify allergies and previous reactions to medications.
- If immunizations are to be given, carefully screen the immunization record (SF 601), located inside the medical record, and/or the international shot record (PHS 731) for dates of previous immunizations and boosters.

3 Verify compatibility of medications if multiple injections are ordered.

4 Ensure that emergency equipment and personnel are available.

⚠ WARNING

Have an emergency tray available for the immediate treatment of serious reactions. Include a constricting band and a syringe containing a 1:1000 solution of epinephrine.

---

5 Wash hands.

6 Identify route of delivery and select the injection site.

○ Route of delivery for medication will be indicated in the order and/or the medication container.

○ Be sure to select the appropriate site for the medication ordered to ensure that the rate of onset and duration are as intended by the provider.

7 Gather equipment (appropriate-size needle, syringe, and type of medication) and prepare medication.

8 Don gloves.

9 Position patient with selected injection site exposed.

CAUTION

All injection sites must be completely exposed prior to injection. Clothing that prevents access to the injection site for visualization, cleaning, and administration of the injection should be removed, and patient privacy ensured by using privacy screens and/or a sheet, towel, or pad to cover the exposed areas.

○ Upper arm: Standing or sitting with arm at side, muscles relaxed, and area completely exposed.

○ Gluteus maximus: Lying face down or leaning forward and supported by a stable object with the weight shifted to the leg that will not be injected. The area is completely exposed.

○ Vastus lateralis: Lying supine or seated. Injection area completely exposed.

It is permissible to use a standing position for injections. However, some patients—even young, healthy soldiers—may experience a vasovagal response to an injection and become dizzy or lose consciousness. The seated or lying positions are therefore preferable.

10 Cleanse the injection site with an alcohol prep pad, beginning in the center of the site. With a circular motion, clean outward for approximately 3 inches.

11 Place alcohol prep pad between the ring finger and little finger of nondominant hand for use after the injection.

Performance Steps for Administration

1 Pull needle cover or cap straight off and dispose of it in a waste receptacle.

2 Isolate the injection site.

○ IM injections: Grasp the muscle mass with thumb and fingers of the nondominant hand and hold it firmly in place.

○ SQ injections: Gently pinch the skin with the thumb and fingers of the nondominant hand and hold it firmly in place.

3 Hold syringe in the dominant hand between the thumb and index finger, and position the needle bevel up and about 0.5 inch from the skin surface.

4 Inject medication.

○ IM injections: Hold syringe at a 90-degree angle to the site and plunge the needle straight into the muscle to the depth of the needle. Hand position will be similar to holding a dart.

○ SQ injections: Hold syringe at a 45-degree angle. Hand position will be similar to holding a pool cue.

5 Release hold on the skin with the nondominant hand.

6 Aspirate by pulling back slightly on the plunger of the syringe.

○ If blood appears, stop the procedure. Dispose of the needle and syringe in a sharps container, prepare a new set, select a different injection site, and begin again.

○ If no blood appears, continue the procedure.

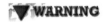

WARNING

Failure to aspirate may cause the medication to be
injected directly into the bloodstream. (This step is not
required for ID injections.)

(7) Using a slow, continuous movement, completely depress the
plunger, injecting the medication.

(8) Place either an alcohol pad or sterile gauze pad lightly over the
injection site and withdraw the needle at the same angle in which
it was inserted.

(9) Gently massage the site, unless this is contraindicated for the
type of medication that has been injected. Place an adhesive
bandage over the injection site.

(10) *Do not recap the needle.* Drop the used needle and syringe into
the sharps container.

(11) Record the administration of the injection on the appropriate
documents.

(12) Either have the patient wait for at least 20 minutes or follow
local SOP and monitor for adverse reactions.

Administering Intradermal Medications
Purpose, Equipment, and Sites for Intradermal (ID) Injections

○ Purpose
  ■ Testing sensitivity to environmental allergens, medications
    (allergy testing)
  ■ Testing for exposure to diseases (e.g., tuberculosis, mumps)
  ■ Evaluation of the immune system (e.g., AIDS and cancer patients)
○ Equipment
  ■ Needle
    • Needle length: 0.25 inch to 0.5 inch
    • Gauge diameter range: 25 to 27
  ■ Tuberculin or other 1.0-mL syringe

- Sites
  - Free of hair, tattoos, and scars
  - *Not* over a vein or bony area
  - Inner forearm: Inner, flat portion (primary injection site for ID)

> **note**
>
> The inner forearm is the preferred site for tuberculin testing and most other ID injections routinely given by the soldier medic.

  - Back of upper arm
  - On the back below the shoulder blades

Preparation and Administration of Intradermal Injections

Performance Steps for Preparation

1 Identify patient.

2 Verify injection.

3 Verify compatibility of medications if multiple injections are ordered.

4 Assure availability of emergency equipment and personnel.

5 Wash hands.

6 Select injection site.

7 Gather equipment and prepare medication.

8 Don gloves.

9 Clean the area with an alcohol prep pad or acetone in a spiral motion; clean outward for approximately 3 inches.

10 Position patient with injection site exposed.

o Inner forearm: Standing, sitting, or supine. Palm up, with the arm relaxed and supported.

o Back of upper arm: Standing or sitting.

o On the back: Prone or seated and leaning forward with body supported by a stable object.

11 Pull the needle cover or cap straight off and dispose of it in a waste receptacle.

12 Using the thumb of the nondominant hand, pull the skin below the injection site downward and hold it taut.

Performance Steps for Administration

1 Position the syringe with the needle bevel up, at a 15- to 20-degree angle to the skin surface.

2 Insert the needle just until the bevel is under the skin surface.

3 Gently release the skin tension held by the nondominant hand.

4 Do not aspirate. Push the plunger slowly forward until all medication has been injected and a wheal (a round or elongated elevation of the skin caused by the injection of fluid under the dermis) appears at the site of the injection.

5 The appearance of a wheal indicates that the medication has entered the area between the intradermal tissues.

o If a wheal does not appear, withdraw the needle completely from the arm at the angle of insertion, dispose of the needle and syringe in a sharps container, prepare a new set, and repeat the procedure in another site.

o If a wheal does appear, continue the procedure.

6 Quickly withdraw the needle at the same angle at which it was inserted.

7 Without applying pressure to the skin surface, cover the injection site with dry sterile gauze.

8 Instruct the patient not to scratch, rub, or wash the injection site.

9 If appropriate, instruct the patient when and where to have the test read in accordance with local SOP.

10 Discard the needle and syringe into the sharps container without recapping the needle.

11 Check the site for bleeding and observe the patient for allergic reactions.

12 Record the procedure on the appropriate form.

CAUTION

If this injection was given to determine sensitivity (PPD), follow local SOP for patient care and instructions for reading of the results in 48 to 72 hours.

Summary

Although the process for administering injections is simple, you must follow the correct procedural steps. Failure to follow the steps may result in the compromise of aseptic technique, improper administration of the medication or immunization, and injury to the patient.

Procedures

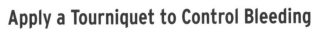

Apply a Tourniquet to Control Bleeding

Performance Steps

 1 Determine if the bleeding is life threatening.

note

If bleeding is profuse, apply direct pressure to the wound with your hand. Do not waste time looking for a dressing.

② Apply direct pressure and a pressure dressing to the wound with an emergency trauma dressing.

○ Apply the dressing, white side down, directly over the wound.
○ Wrap the tail around the limb and run the tail through the plastic pressure device. Reverse the tail while applying pressure and continue to wrap the remainder of the wrap around the extremity, continuing to apply pressure directly over the wound. Secure the plastic fastening clip to the last turn of the wrap.
○ Check the dressing to make sure that it is applied firmly enough to prevent slipping without causing a tourniquet-like effect.

③ Apply a tourniquet if the wound continues to bleed.

> **CAUTION**
>
> In combat while under enemy fire, a tourniquet is the primary means to control bleeding. It allows the individual or his or her battle buddy to quickly control life-threatening hemorrhage until the casualty can be moved out of the firefight.

○ Place the tourniquet a minimum of 2 inches above the wound or amputation. The tourniquet should be a minimum of 2 inches wide.
○ Wrap the cravat around the limb and tie a half-knot.
○ Place some type of windlass device (e.g., a stick, bayonet scabbard, flashlight) on top of the half-knot, and tie a full knot on top of the windlass device.
○ Twist the windlass device until it tightens enough to stop the bleeding.
○ Secure the windlass device so that it will not loosen or unwind.
○ Mark the casualty with a "T" on the forehead to alert others of the tourniquet.

④ Loosen the tourniquet in accordance with the following guidelines:

○ Once the tactical situation allows and more time is available without hostile fire.
○ Consider loosening the tourniquet if it has been in place for less than 6 hours.
○ Once the tourniquet is loosened, use direct pressure or pressure dressings to control the bleeding. This will allow the preservation of the extremity and prevent amputation if the tourniquet is left in place for prolonged periods.
○ If unable to control hemorrhage by other methods, tighten the tourniquet until bleeding stops.

note

If you are unable to control hemorrhage with any method other than a tourniquet, it is better to sacrifice a limb than to lose a life due to uncontrolled hemorrhage.

5 Assess the need for evacuation.

6 Reassess injury to ensure that bleeding has been controlled.

7 If the source of bleeding was due to a traumatic amputation:

o Wrap the amputated part in a clean cloth or sterile dressing (if available).
o Wrap or bag the amputated part in plastic.
o Label the plastic bag with the patient's information.
o Transport the amputated part in a cool container (if available) with the patient.

CAUTION

Do not place the amputated part directly on ice. Do not submerge it directly in water. Do not allow the part to freeze.

Apply a Combat Application Tourniquet

A Combat Application Tourniquet (**Figure 19**) is the tourniquet of choice for the following reasons:

o Controls bleeding
o Lightweight
o Easy to use

Performance Steps

The method for applying a Combat Application Tourniquet is detailed in the following steps (see **Figure 20**).

1 Place the wounded extremity through the loop of the self-adhering band.

2 Place tourniquet above the injury site.

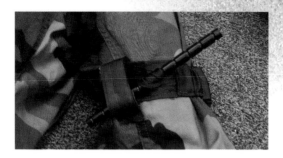

Figure 19   Combat Application Tourniquet.

3 Pull the free-running end of the self-adhering band tight and securely fasten it back on itself.

4 Adhere completely around the band until the clip is reached.

5 Twist the windlass rod until the bleeding has stopped.

6 Lock the windlass rod in place with the windlass clip.

7 For small extremities, continue to adhere the self-adhering band around the extremity and over the windlass rod.

8 Grasp the windlass strap, pull it tight, and adhere it to the Velcro on the windlass clip.

9 The Combat Application Tourniquet is now ready for transport.

note

The friction adaptor buckle is not necessary for proper Combat Application Tourniquet application to an arm. It must be used with two hands when applying to a leg.

note

Large extremity application: To use, wrap the self-adhering band through the friction adaptor buckle. This prevents the strap from loosening during transport.

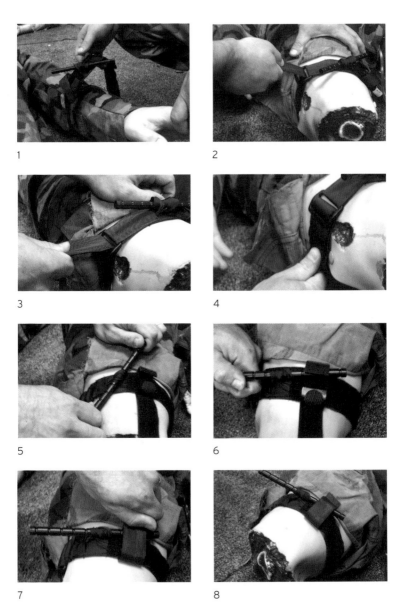

Figure 20 Steps for applying a Combat Application Tourniquet.

Apply an Emergency Trauma Dressing

1 Uncover the wound unless clothing is stuck to the wound.

2 Apply the casualty's emergency trauma dressing.

○ Apply the dressing, white side down, directly over the wound.
○ Wrap the elastic bandage around the limb or body part.
○ Insert elastic bandage into the pressure bar.
○ Tighten elastic bandage.
○ Pull back, forcing the pressure bar down onto the pad.
○ Wrap the elastic bandage tightly over the pressure bar and wrap over all edges of the pad.
○ Secure the hooking ends of the closure bar into the elastic bandage.

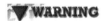 **WARNING**

The emergency trauma dressing should not have a tourniquet-like effect. The dressing must be loosened if the skin beyond the injury becomes cool, blue, or numb.

○ Check to make sure that the dressing is secured firmly enough to prevent slipping without causing a tourniquet-like effect.

3 Apply manual pressure and elevate the casualty's arm or leg to reduce bleeding, if necessary.

○ Apply firm manual pressure over the dressing for 5 to 10 minutes.
○ Elevate the injured part above the level of the heart unless a fracture is suspected and has not been splinted.

Administer Morphine

1 Verify the "five rights" of medication administration.

○ Right patient: Verify that the casualty does not have any contraindications that preclude the use of morphine.
○ Right medication: Check to ensure the medication you are about to administer is correct.

○ Right dosage
  ■ IV morphine dosage
    • Administer an initial dose of 5 mg IV (*slow* push over 4 to 5 minutes). Morphine given via IV should be diluted in 5 mL of sterile water for injection or with normal saline prior to usage.
    • When morphine is given intravenously, repeat doses may be given every 10 minutes. Most adults will experience pain relief at a total dose of 10 to 20 mg, although higher doses may be needed.
  ■ IM morphine dosage
    • Load the prefilled cartridge into the injector device (usually at a dose of 5 or 10 mg). If the medic is not giving the full 10-mg amount to the casualty, place the unused portion in another syringe (if possible) to utilize the full amount of morphine later. In other words, don't waste medication.
    • The U.S. military utilizes auto-injectors. The dosage is usually 1 auto-injector (10 mg).
○ Right time: Check the casualty's forehead and Field Medical Card (FMC) to see when the last dose was administered and how much was given.
○ Right route: Morphine comes in multiple strengths and routes of administration (oral, intramuscular, subcutaneous, and intravenous injection). In combat situations, the IV route is the preferred method of administration due to a more rapid pain response than achieved with the more traditional IM methods.

2 Load the prefilled cartridge into the injector device.

○ Insert the cartridge into the body and guard assembly.
○ Align the finger grip assembly notches and snap into place.

3 Lock the cartridge into the injector device by turning the plunger rod until the plunger is securely in place.

4 Place the casualty in a supine position.

> **note** ─────────────────────────────────
>
> Once morphine has been administered, the casualty is considered nonambulatory.

5 Select the site for an intramuscular injection.

○ Deltoid muscle
○ Buttocks
○ Outer thigh

6 Administer the injection.

7 If using an auto-injector, complete the following steps.

○ Remove the safety cap.
○ Place purple end on outer thigh and press firmly to deliver the dosage.

8 Monitor for adverse reactions.

> **note**
>
> The most common adverse reaction is severe respiratory depression. The casualty may require assisted ventilations.

○ If morphine overdose is suspected, administer naloxone (Narcan).
- The dose of Narcan given is 0.4 mg to 2 mg *slow* IV push over 1 to 2 minutes. Narcan may need to be repeated three to four times. Some authorities recommend up to 10-20 mg of Narcan to treat suspected morphine overdose.
- An immediate positive response is usually seen when giving Narcan for morphine poisoning. The duration of action for Narcan is 1 to 2 hours.
- Narcan's effect may wear off earlier than the morphine, permitting the patient to lapse back into respiratory depression. Continuous monitoring of a patient being given Narcan to counteract morphine toxicity is crucial. After every dose of Narcan given, thoroughly reassess the patient.
- Narcan should be adjusted according to the patient's respiratory status, not the level of consciousness.
- Document every dose given and the time given on the casualty's FMC.

9 Write the letter "M" and the time of injection on the casualty's forehead.

10 Document morphine doses on DD Form 1380.

Insert a Nasopharyngeal Airway

Performance Steps

1 Place the casualty supine with the head in a neutral position.

CAUTION

Do not use the nasopharyngeal airway if there is clear fluid (cerebrospinal fluid) coming from the ears or nose. This may indicate a skull fracture.

2 Select the appropriate size of airway using one of the following methods:

o Measure the airway from the patient's nostril to the earlobe.
o Measure the airway from the patient's nostril to the angle of the jaw.

note

Choosing the proper length ensures appropriate diameter. Standard adult sizes are 34, 32, 30, and 28 French.

3 Lubricate the tube with a water-based lubricant.

CAUTION

Do not use a petroleum-based or non-water-based lubricant. These substances can cause damage to the tissues lining the nasal cavity and pharynx, thus increasing the risk for infection.

4 Insert the airway.

o Push the tip of the nose upward gently.
o Position the tube so that the bevel of the airway faces toward the septum.

note

Most nasopharyngeal airways are designed to be placed in the right nostril.

o Insert the airway into the nostril and advance it until the flange rests against the nostril.

CAUTION

Never force the airway into the patient's nostril. If resistance is met, pull the tube out and attempt to insert it in the other nostril.

Insert a Combitube

1 Oxygenate the casualty.

o Instruct the assistant to hyperventilate the casualty for 30 seconds using the bag-valve-mask (BVM) device.

2 Prepare the Combitube.

o Inspect the tube for breaks or cracks.
o Attach the large syringe to the pharyngeal (proximal) cuff and inflate it with 100 cc of air. Check for leaks and then deflate completely.
o Attach the small syringe to the tracheal (distal) cuff and inflate it with 15 cc of air. Check for leaks and then deflate completely.

> **note**
>
> If a leak is present, replace the tube.

3 Put on gloves.

4 Kneel just above the casualty's head, facing the casualty's feet.

> **note**
>
> If the casualty's neck has been hyperextended to open the airway, return it to a neutral position.

5 Insert the tube.

o Lift the jaw and tongue straight upward without hyperextending the neck.
o Pass the tube gently but firmly, following the pharyngeal curvature, until the teeth are between the two black lines on the tube.

> **CAUTION**
>
> Do not force the tube at any time. If the tube does not insert easily, withdraw it and retry. Hyperventilate the patient between each attempt.

o Use the large syringe to inflate the no. 1 blue pharyngeal cuff with 100 cc of air. The device will seat itself in the posterior pharynx behind the hard palate.

o Use the small syringe to inflate the no. 2 white distal cuff with 15 cc of air.

6 Ventilate the casualty and check tube placement.

o Attach the BVM device to the esophageal connector (blue no. 1 tube).

o Attempt to ventilate and listen for the presence of breath sounds in the lungs and absence of sounds from the epigastrium.

o If there is an absence of breath sounds and presence of sounds in the epigastrium, the tube is in the trachea.

o Attach the BVM device to the tracheal connector (white no. 2 tube) and ventilate the casualty.

o Listen for the presence of breath sounds, and absence of gastric sounds.

o Continue to ventilate the casualty every 3 to 5 seconds.

7 Remove the Combitube if the casualty regains consciousness or regains a gag reflex.

o Oxygenate the casualty with two slow breaths.

o Turn the casualty to one side.

o Deflate the large no. 1 tube first, and then the smaller no. 2 tube.

o Withdraw the tube in one quick motion, following the curve of the pharynx.

o Immediately clear the casualty's airway of any vomitus.

> **note** ————————————————————————
>
> Suction should be readily available when removing a Combitube.

Perform a Cricothyroidotomy

Performance Steps

CAUTION

Consider only casualties with a total upper airway obstruction, casualties with inhalation burns, or casualties with massive maxillofacial trauma who cannot be ventilated by other means for a surgical cricothyroidotomy.

1 Gather cricothyroidotomy kit or minimum essential equipment.

> **note**
>
> Because of the need for speed, every medic should have an easily accessible cricothyroidotomy kit that contains all required items. Do not delay getting an airway established for lack of nonessential equipment.

- Cutting instrument: Number 10 or 15 scalpel or knife blade.
- Airway tube: Endotracheal tube (ETT), tracheotomy tube, or any noncollapsible tube that will allow enough airflow to maintain oxygen saturation.

> **note**
>
> In a field setting, an ETT is preferred because it is easy to secure. Use a size 6 or 7 ETT, and ensure the cuff will hold air.

2 Hyperextend the casualty's neck.

> ▼ **WARNING**
>
> Do not hyperextend the casualty's neck if a cervical injury is suspected.

- Place the casualty in the supine position.
- Place a rolled-up blanket or poncho under the casualty's neck or between the shoulder blades to hyperextend the neck.

3 Put on gloves.

4 Locate the cricothyroid membrane.

- Place a finger of the nondominant hand on the thyroid cartilage (Adam's apple), and slide the finger down to the cricoid cartilage.
- Palpate for the soft cricothyroid membrane below the thyroid cartilage and just above the cricoid cartilage.
- Slide the index finger down into the depression between the thyroid and cricoid cartilage.
- Prepare the skin over the membrane with povidone iodine.

5 With a cutting instrument in the dominant hand, make a 1.5-inch vertical incision over the cricothyroid membrane.

note

The reason for a vertical incision rather than a horizontal incision is that a vertical incision will allow visualization of the cricothyroid membrane but keep the scalpel blade away from the lateral aspect of the neck. This is important because of the large blood vessels located in the lateral areas of the neck. This technique will help eliminate costly mistakes.

CAUTION

Do not cut the cricothyroid membrane with this incision.

6 Relocate the cricothyroid membrane by touch and sight.

7 Stabilize the larynx with one hand and cut through the cricothyroid membrane.

note

A rush of air may be felt through the opening.

o If using a no. 10 or 15 scalpel blade, make a 0.5-inch horizontal incision through the elastic tissue of the cricothyroid membrane.

8 Insert the tip of an 18-gauge needle formed into a hook through the opening; hook the cricoid cartilage and lift to stabilize the opening.

9 Insert the end of the ETT or tracheotomy tube through the opening and toward the lungs. The tube should be in the trachea and directed toward the lungs. Inflate the cuff with 5 to 10 cc of air.

note

Do not advance the tube more than 2 to 3 inches, because this could result in the intubation of only the right main stem bronchus.

10 Check for air exchange and placement of the tube.

○ Air exchange
  ■ Listen and feel for air passing in and out of the tube.
  ■ Look for bilateral rise and fall of the chest.
○ Placement of the tube
  ■ If there are bilateral breath sounds and bilateral rise and fall of the chest, the tube is properly placed and may be secured.
  ■ If there is unilateral rise and fall of the chest, absent or unilateral breath sounds, epigastric gurgling, air escaping from the casualty's mouth or from around the tube, or air infiltrating into the tissues of the neck or chest, the tube is improperly placed and corrective action must be initiated immediately.
    • Unilateral breath sounds and unilateral rise and fall of the chest indicate that the tube is past the carina. Deflate the cuff, retract the tube 1 to 2 inches, and recheck air exchange and placement.
    • Air coming out of the casualty's mouth indicates the tube is pointed away from the lungs. Remove the tube, reinsert, and recheck for air exchange and placement.
    • Any other problem is indicative of the tube not being in the trachea. Remove the tube, reinsert, and recheck for air exchange and placement.

11 If the tube is correctly placed but the casualty is not breathing, direct someone to perform rescue breathing, based on the tactical situation.

○ Connect the tube to a BVM device (with oxygen if available), and ventilate the casualty at the rate of 20 breaths/min.
○ If no BVM is available, have someone perform mouth-to-tube resuscitation at 20 breaths/min.
○ Once rescue breathing has started, secure the tube, using tape, cloth ties, or other measures.

12 Apply a dressing to further protect the tube and incision by using one of the following techniques.

○ Cut two 4 × 4-inch or 4 × 8-inch gauze pads halfway through. Place them on opposite sides of the tube so that the tube comes up through the cut, and the gauze overlaps. Tape securely.
○ Apply a sterile dressing under the casualty's tube by making a V-shaped fold in a 4 × 8-inch gauze pad and placing it under the edge of the cannula to prevent irritation to the casualty. Tape securely.

13 Monitor casualty's respirations on a regular basis.

○ Reassess air exchange and placement every time the casualty is moved.
○ Assist respirations if respiratory rate falls below 12 or rises above 20 breaths/min.

Perform Needle Chest Decompression

Performance Steps

> **note**
>
> Pneumothorax is defined as the presence of air within the chest cavity. Air may enter the chest cavity either from the lungs (through a rupture or laceration) or from the outside (through a sucking chest wound). Trapped air in the chest cavity under pressure, called a tension pneumothorax, compresses the lung beneath it. Unrelieved pressure will push and compress the contents of the chest in the opposite direction, away from the side of the tension pneumothorax. This, in turn, will prevent the heart from filling with blood and beating correctly and the good lung from providing adequate respirations.

CAUTION

This procedure would *only* be performed if the casualty has a penetrating wound to the chest and increasing trouble breathing.

1 Locate the insertion site. Locate the second intercostal space approximately 2 fingerbreadths below the clavicle (between the second and third ribs) at the midclavicular line (approximately in line with the nipple) on the same side of the patient's chest as the penetrating wound.

2 Insert a large-bore (10- to 14-gauge 3-inch) needle and catheter unit.

○ Firmly insert the needle into the skin over the top of the third rib into the second intercostal space until the chest cavity has been penetrated, as evidenced by feeling a "pop" as the needle enters the chest cavity. A hiss of escaping air under pressure should be heard.

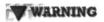

WARNING

Proper positioning of the needle is essential to avoid puncturing blood vessels and/or nerves. Blood vessels and nerves run along the bottom of each rib.

3 Withdraw the needle while holding the catheter still. Secure the catheter to the chest wall using tape.

4 The casualty's respiration should improve. Monitor the casualty until medical care arrives.

Insert a Chest Tube

Performance Steps

1 Assess the casualty.

- If necessary, open the airway.
- Ensure adequate respiration and assist as necessary.
- Provide supplemental oxygen, if available.
- Connect the casualty to a pulse oximeter, if available.
- Initiate an IV.

2 Prepare the casualty.

- Place the casualty in the supine position.
- Raise the arm on the affected side above the casualty's head.
- Select the insertion site at the anterior axillary line over the fourth or fifth intercostal space.
- Clean the site with povidone iodine (Betadine) solution.
- Put on sterile gloves.
- Drape the area.
- Liberally infiltrate the area with 1% lidocaine solution.

3 Insert the tube.

- Make a 2- to 3-cm transverse incision over the selected site and extend it down to the intercostal muscles.

> **note**
>
> The skin incision should be 1 to 2 cm below the inter-space through which the tube will be placed.

o Insert the Kelly forceps through the intercostal muscles in the next intercostal space.
o Puncture the parietal pleura with the tip of the forceps and slightly enlarge the hole by opening the clamp 1.5 to 2 cm.

> **CAUTION**
>
> Avoid puncturing the lung. Always use the superior margin of the rib to avoid the intercostal nerves and vessels.

o Immediately insert a gloved finger in the incision to clear any adhesions, clots, etc.
o Grasp the tip of the chest tube with Kelly forceps. Insert the tip of the tube in the incision as you withdraw your finger.
o Advance the tube until the last side hole is 2.5 to 5 cm inside the chest wall.
o Connect the end of the tube to a one-way drainage valve (e.g., Heimlich valve).
o Secure the tube using the suture materials.
o Apply an occlusive dressing to the site.
o Radiograph the chest to confirm placement, if available.

④ Reassess the casualty.

o Check for bilateral breath sounds.
o Monitor and record vital signs every 15 minutes.

⑤ Document the procedure.

Initiate an Intraosseous Infusion

Performance Steps

The following steps outline the correct procedure for inserting the F.A.S.T.1 intraosseous infusion system (see **Figure 21**).

① Prepare the site.

o Undo or cut shirt to expose the sternum.
o Identify the sternal notch.
o Use aseptic technique to prepare the site.

② Place the target patch.

o Remove the top half of the backing (labeled "Remove 1") from the patch.
o Locate the sternal notch using your index finger.

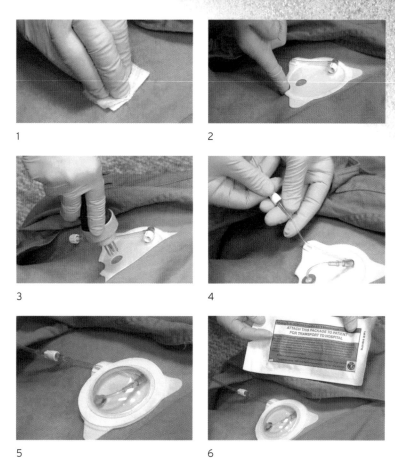

Figure 21

○ Holding your index finger perpendicular to the skin, align the locating notch in the target patch with the sternal notch, keeping your index finger perpendicular.

○ Verify that the target zone (circular hole) on the patch is directly over the patient's midline.

○ Secure the top half of the patch to the body by pressing firmly downward on the patch, engaging the adhesive.

○ Remove the remaining backing (labeled "Remove 2") and secure patch to the patient.

○ Verify correct patch placement by checking the alignment of the locating notch with the patient's sternal notch and making sure the target zone is over the midline of the patient's body.

3 Insert introducer.

○ Remove the sharps cap from the introducer.
○ Place bone probe cluster needles in the target zone of the target patch, and ensure that all the bone probe needles are within the target zone.
○ Hold the introducer perpendicular to the skin of the patient to ensure proper functioning of the depth-control mechanism.
○ Pressing straight along the introducer axis, with hand and elbow in line, push with firm, constant force until a distinct release is heard and felt.

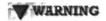 **WARNING**

> Apply the force perpendicular to the skin and along the long axis of the introducer. Avoid extreme force and twisting and jabbing motions.

○ After the release, expose the infusion tube by gently withdrawing the introducer along the same path used to insert it (perpendicular to the skin). The stylet supports will fall away.
○ Locate the orange sharps plug, and place it on a flat surface with the foam facing up. Keep both hands behind the needles, and push the bone probe cluster straight into the foam. After the sharps plug has been engaged and the sharps are safely covered, reattach the clear sharps cap to the introducer. This completes the dual sharps protection.
○ Dispose of the introducer using contaminated sharps protocols.

4 Connect infusion tube.

○ Connect the infusion tube to the right-angle female connector on the target patch.

> **note**
>
> This connection is a slip luer.

○ Optional step: Verify correct placement of infusion tube by attaching the enclosed syringe to the straight female connector and withdrawing marrow into the infusion tube.
○ Attach the straight female connector to the source of fluids or drugs. Fluid can now flow to the site.

5 Secure the protector dome.

○ Place the protector dome directly over the target patch and press down firmly to engage the Velcro fastening. Ensure that the infusion tubing and the right-angle female connector are contained under the dome.

○ The dome can be removed by holding the patch against the skin and peeling back the dome Velcro.

6 Attach the remover package.

○ Attach the remover package to the patient for transport.

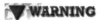**WARNING**

The remover package must be transported with the patient. It will be used later to remove the F.A.S.T.1 system.

───────────────────────────────────────

note ──────────────────────────────────

Do not breach the packaging, because the remover is sterile.

───────────────────────────────────────

7 Record all treatment on the Field Medical Card.

Remove an Intraosseous Infusion
Performance Steps

The following steps outline the correct procedure for removing the F.A.S.T.1 intraosseous infusion system (see **Figure 22**).

1 Remove the dome.

○ Remove the protector dome from the patch by peeling the Velcro ring away from the patch.

note ──────────────────────────────────

Make sure one hand is holding the patch against the patient's skin while the other hand peels the dome Velcro up so that the patch does not come away from the skin during the process.

───────────────────────────────────────

2 Disconnect the infusion tube.

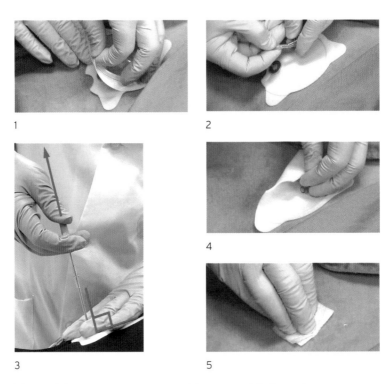

Figure 22   Removing the F.A.S.T.1 intraosseous infusion system.

○ Ensure that the clamp controlling the IV fluid flow is turned off.
○ Disconnect the IV line from the straight female connector tube on the patch.
○ Disconnect the infusion tube from the right-angle female connector on the patch.

3   Remove the infusion tube.

▼ WARNING

Do *not* pull on the infusion tube to remove it.

○ Open the remover package while maintaining aseptic technique.
○ Remove the tubing protecting the remover tip.
○ Insert the remover into infusion tube while holding the infusion tube straight out (90 degrees) from the patient.

- Advance the remover, and turn it clockwise until it stops. This will engage the threads in the proximal tip of the infusion tube.
- Use one hand to press down lightly on the target patch, and the other to pull the remover straight out to dislodge the infusion tube. Hold the remover by the T-shaped knob. Do *not* hold the luer or tubing. If the remover disengages from the infusion tube without removing it, make another attempt.

Make sure that you pull the remover in the direction perpendicular to the infusion site to avoid bending of the remover tip.

4 Remove the target patch.

- Gently peel the target patch away from the patient and discard the patch.

5 Dress the infusion site.

- Apply pressure to the infusion site.
- Reassess to check bleeding from site.
- Dress the infusion site using aseptic technique.
- Dispose of the remover and infusion tube using contaminated sharps protocols.

Suture a Minor Laceration

Performance Steps

1 Prepare the site.

- Expose the area to be sutured.
- Gently scrub the site with an antiseptic solution using circular motions for a minimum of 5 minutes.

note

Use ample pressure to remove dirt and microorganisms.

- Irrigate the wound with a copious amount of normal saline at a low pressure.
- Dry the site using sterile gauze pads.

2 Anesthetize the area.

o Cryoanesthesia
- Apply a moistened ice cube to the skin for about 5 minutes.
- Spray the area with commercial refrigerants, as directed.

o Topical applications
- Apply the agent directly to the mucous membrane, serous surface, or the open wound.
- Slightly saturate a gauze pad with the appropriate agent and place it on the wound for 5 to 10 minutes.
- Check the area for tissue blanching, which indicates adequate anesthesia.

> **note**
>
> Often topical application is suboptimal for suture placement.

o Simple infiltration
- Ensure the casualty does not have an allergy to the agent.
- Using a needle and syringe, draw up an adequate amount of 1% lidocaine.

> **note**
>
> Lidocaine with epinephrine is never used on the tip of the nose, ears, fingers, toes, or genitalia due to vasoconstriction.

- Enter directly into the dermis through the laceration.
- Aspirate prior to injecting the solution to ensure the needle is not in a vessel. (If blood returns into the syringe, withdraw, change the needle, and try a new site.)
- Slowly inject solution beneath the skin surface, raising a wheal in the area to be anesthetized.
- Repeat steps, depending on the size of the laceration.

3 Select the method of closure.

o Skin adhesive
- Hold the wound edges together and slightly everted with tissue forceps (**Figure 23**).
- Apply adhesive with the applicator tip by lightly wiping along the long axis of the wound.

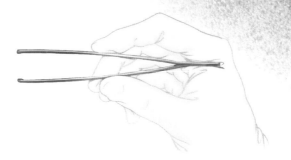

Figure 23 Hold the forceps like a writing utensil. The forceps is used to support the skin edges when you place the sutures. Be careful not to grab the skin too hard, or you will leave marks that can lead to scarring. Ideally, you should grab the dermis or subcutaneous tissue—not the skin—with the forceps, but this technique takes practice. For suturing skin, try to use forceps with teeth, which are little pointed edges at the end of the forceps.

> **note**
>
> Three to four thin layers should be applied successively. Avoid droplets or a single thick layer.

- Hold the wound edges together for approximately 1 minute.
- Instruct the casualty not to apply ointment or dressing to the wound.
○ Steri-Strips
  - Apply benzoin to a 2- to 3-cm area beyond the wound edges. Do not allow benzoin to enter the wound.
  - Using forceps, attach the strip to the skin on one side and then pull it across the wound to close the wound edges.
  - Start in the center and progress toward each end. Leave some space between individual strips.
  - Instruct the casualty not to get the area wet.
○ Staples
  - Hold the wound edges together with tissue forceps.
  - Place the stapling device gently against the skin surface.
  - Slowly squeeze the trigger.
  - Evenly place only the necessary amount of staples to close the wound.

note
There is little to no benefit to locally infiltrating an area for placement of one to two staples. The anesthetic causes more discomfort than the procedure.

o Suture
   ■ Select the proper size and type of material.
   ■ Check for adequate anesthesia by grasping the wound edges with tissue forceps. Note if the casualty can feel pain.
   ■ Grasp the needle with the needle holder (**Figures 24 and 25**) about one half to one third the distance from where the suture is attached.
   ■ Hold the needle holder in the palm, using the index finger for fine control.
   ■ Enter the skin at approximately a 90-degree angle on the far side of the wound, and exit on the near side.

note
You should enter and exit the skin about 2 mm from the edge. Entry and exit points should be directly across from each other.

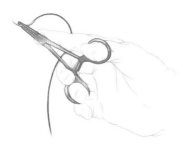

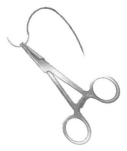

Figure 24   The needle holder and scissors are handled similarly. For maximal control, place the tips of your thumb and ring finger into the rings of the instrument. Your thumb does most of the work to open and close the instrument.

Figure 25   The needle should be held in the jaws of the needle holder at its midpoint (where the curve of the needle is relatively flat). This technique prevents you from bending the needle as it passes through the tissues.

- Pull the suture through the wound until approximately a 2-cm tail remains on the far side of wound.
- Hold the end of the suture attached to the needle in the nondominant hand.
- Hold the needle holder in the dominant hand.
- Loop the suture twice around the needle holder.
- Grasp the free end of the suture with the blades of the needle holder.
- Cross the hands so that the hand holding the swagged end is on the far side and the hand holding the needle holder and free end is on the near side of the wound.
- Pull upward on the suture ends when clinching the first throw.
- Adjust the tension of the first throw so that the wound edges come together snugly but not tightly.
- For the second throw of the knot, the needle end is on the far side of the wound and the free end is on the near side (see **Figure 26**).
- Hold the needle end of the suture in the nondominant hand and lay the needle holder on top.
- Loop the suture only once around the needle holder.
- Grasp the free ends with the blades of the holder.
- Cross the hands so that the sutures smoothly intertwine.
- Cinch down the throw.

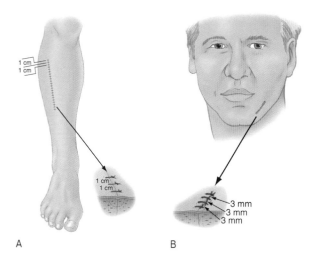

A   B

Figure 26   Placing the sutures. A: For most areas of the body, except the face, the sutures should be placed in the skin 3 to 4 mm from the wound edge and 5 to 10 mm apart. B: Sutures placed on the face should be approximately 2 to 3 mm from the skin edge and 3 to 5 mm apart.

CAUTION

Take care not to cinch down too tightly on the second throw
because the tightness will be transmitted to the wound.

- Pull the knot to the side so that it will not directly overlie the laceration.
- The pattern of looping the suture around the holder on alternate
  sides of the wound is repeated until the desired number of throws
  is completed.
- Cut the ends of the suture material to a length of approximately
  3 to 5 cm.

4 Apply antibiotic ointment to the site.

5 Apply a sterile dressing to the site.

6 Document the procedure.

Placing Sutures

Start on the side of the wound opposite and farthest from you to ensure
that you are always sewing toward yourself. By sewing toward yourself,
the suturing process is made easier from a biomechanical standpoint.

note

Do not drive yourself crazy by placing too many sutures.

- Simple sutures
  - Indication: This technique is the easiest to perform. It is used for
    most skin suturing.
  - Technique
    - Start from the outside of the skin, go through the epidermis into the
      subcutaneous tissue from one side, then enter the subcutaneous tis-
      sue on the opposite side and come out the epidermis above.
    - To evert the edges, the needle tip should enter at a 90-degree
      angle to the skin (**Figure 27**). Then turn your wrist to get the
      needle through the tissues.
    - You can use simple sutures for a continuous or interrupted clo-
      sure (**Figure 28**).
- Interrupted sutures
  - Interrupted sutures are individually placed and tied.

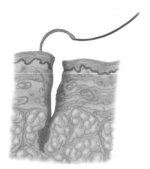

Figure 27 The needle tip should enter the tissues perpendicular to the skin. Once the needle tip has penetrated the top layers of the skin, twist your wrist so that the needle passes through the subcutaneous tissue and then comes out into the wound. This technique helps to ensure that skin edges will evert.

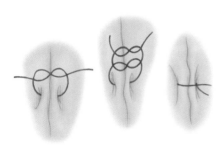

Figure 28 A simple suture.

- They are the technique of choice if you are worried about the cleanliness of the wound. If the wound looks like it is becoming infected, a few sutures can be removed easily without disrupting the entire closure.
- Interrupted sutures can be used in all areas but may take longer to place than a continuous suture.
○ Continuous closure
  - Place the sutures again and again without tying each individual suture.
  - If the wound is very clean and it is easy to bring the edges together, a continuous closure is adequate and quick to perform.
  - Continuous closure is the technique of choice to help stop bleeding from the skin edges, which is important, for example, in a scalp laceration.

Insert a Urinary Catheter

Performance Steps

1 Clean the urinary meatus with the prepared cotton balls or swabs.

note ──

Cotton balls should be held with forceps.

──

o Females
  ■ Gently spread the labia open with the nondominant hand.

  note ──────────────────────────────────────

  This hand is now considered contaminated.

  ──

  • Place the thumb and forefinger between the labia minora.
  • Separate the labia and pull up slightly.
  ■ With the dominant hand, clean the labia with cotton balls or
    swabs, moving from the clitoris toward the anus.
  ■ Use a cotton ball or swab to clean down the center, directly over
    the urinary meatus.
  ■ Keep the labia spread throughout the remainder of the procedure.
o Males
  ■ Support the penis with the nondominant hand.

  note ──────────────────────────────────────

  This hand is now considered contaminated.

  ──

  ■ With the dominant hand, clean the penis with a cotton ball or
    swab, moving in a circular motion from the urinary meatus toward
    the base of the penis.
  ■ Repeat the procedure, using a second and third cotton ball or swab.

②   Lubricate the catheter.

o Pick up the catheter with the dominant hand about 4 inches from the tip.
o Keep the distal end of the catheter coiled in the palm of the hand.
o Apply lubricant to the catheter tip.

③   Instruct the patient to relax and breathe through the mouth.

④   Insert the catheter.

o Female
  ■ Gently insert the catheter into the urethra about 2 to 3 inches
    until resistance is met.
  ■ Continue to advance the catheter until urine begins to flow (about
    2 to 3 inches further).

- Release the labia and hold the catheter securely with the nondominant hand.
- Place the distal end of the catheter in the collection basin.

note

If the vagina is inadvertently catheterized, do not remove the catheter. Assemble new equipment and repeat the procedure. Leaving the first catheter in place temporarily will prevent catheterizing the vagina a second time.

○ Male
- Draw the penis upward and forward to a 60- to 90-degree angle to the legs.
- Gently insert the catheter into the urethra, advancing it about 7 to 8 inches or until resistance is felt.
- Continue to advance the catheter until urine begins to flow (about 2 to 3 inches further).
- Lower the penis and hold the catheter securely with the nondominant hand, resting the hand on the patient's pubis for support.
- Place the distal end of the catheter in the collection basin.

note

With some commercially prepared catheterization kits, the catheter is preconnected to the drainage tubing of the collecting bag.

5 Obtain a urine specimen, if ordered.

○ Place the sterile specimen container from the kit into the collection basin.
○ Pinch the catheter with the nondominant hand to stop urine flow.
○ With the dominant hand, pick up the distal end of the catheter and hold it over the specimen container.
○ Release the pinch and allow sufficient urine to drain into the specimen container (about 30 cc).
○ Repinch the catheter, place the distal end into the collection basin, and release the pinch, allowing the urine to flow.
○ Place the lid on the specimen container and set it aside.

note

If using a commercial kit with the catheter and drainage set preconnected, do not disconnect the catheter to obtain a specimen. Obtain the specimen from the drainage bag at the end of the procedure. The first specimen taken from a new sterile drainage set is considered sterile.

6 Inflate the balloon if an indwelling catheter has been inserted.

○ Inflate the balloon with the water in the prefilled syringe.

note

If the balloon is difficult to inflate, advance the catheter another 0.5 to 1 inch to ensure that the catheter tip is fully within the bladder.

○ Tug gently on the catheter to ensure that the balloon is fully inflated and seated in the bladder.

○ Remove the syringe from the catheter using a twisting motion.

7 Attach the distal end of the catheter to the drainage tubing of the collection set, if not preconnected by the manufacturer.

8 Remove the drapes and gloves.

9 Tape the catheter in place.

○ Female: Tape to the inner thigh.

○ Male: Tape to the abdomen or inner thigh.

note

The penis may be positioned up or down (facing the patient's head or feet), depending upon the patient's diagnosis, the physician's order, and/or the patient's comfort preference.

10 Secure the drainage bag to the side of the bed on the bottom of the bed frame.

CAUTION

Do not secure the drainage bag to the bed siderails or loop the drainage tubing over or through the siderails.

11 Reposition the patient.

12 Dispose of the used equipment and clean the area.

> **note**
>
> Destroy the syringe and dispose of it in accordance with local SOP for infectious waste.

13 Report and record the procedure.

Prepare an Aid Bag

Performance Steps

> **note**
>
> The contents of the aid bag will be based on the type and length of the mission and the skill level of the combat medic. There is no standard packing list for an aid bag.

1 Determine the type of aid bag available:

- M-5 aid bag
- Blackhawk aid bag
- London Bridge aid bag
- Skedco aid bag
- Others

2 Contents (based on the skill level of individual medic)

- Airway supplies
  - Nasopharyngeal airways
  - Oropharyngeal airways
  - Combitube kit
  - Surgical cricothyroidotomy kit

- Breathing supplies
  - Vaseline gauze pads (occlusive dressing)
  - Asherman chest seal
  - 10- to 14-gauge 2.5- to 3-inch needle catheter unit (needle chest decompression)
- Circulation supplies
  - Kerlix
  - Emergency trauma dressings (Israeli bandage)
  - Cravats
  - Tourniquets
  - Improvised windlass devices (7 to 10 tongue depressors wrapped in duct tape)
  - IV infusion sets
  - IV fluids
  - F.A.S.T.1 sternal intraosseous infusion device
  - Constricting band
  - Alcohol pads
  - Iodine pads
  - Tegaderm dressings
  - 18-gauge IV catheters
  - Saline locks
  - Hemostatic bandages (chitosan)
- Fracture supplies
  - Sam splints
  - Miscellaneous splints
  - Ace wraps (2, 4, and 6 inch)
- Antibiotics
  - Gatifloxacin tablets, 400 mg
  - Cefotetan, 2-g injection
- Pain medications
  - Morphine Tubex injectors, 10 mg/mL
  - Toradol 10 mg
  - Acetaminophen tablets, 500 mg
- Nuclear, biological, and chemical (NBC) medications
  - NAAK (nerve agent antidote kit) injectors
  - CANA (convalescent antidote for nerve agent) injectors
- Miscellaneous supplies
  - Large abdominal pad
  - Tape nylon (1-, 2-, and 3-inch size)
  - Gauze pads, 4 × 4 inch
  - Gauze pads, 2 × 2 inch

- Eye pads
- Cotton-tipped applicators
- Band-Aids
- ENT kit
- Stethoscope
- Burn packs
- Surgilube
- Tincture of benzoin
- Exam gloves
- Adjustable C-collar
- Field Medical Card
- Bandage scissors
- Needles (various sizes)
- Syringes (various sizes)
- Chemlites
- Space blanket
- Oral hydration solution packs
- Tongue depressors
- Miscellaneous medications based on medical officer's determination

Conduct Medical Resupply

Initial Medical Resupply

- During deployment, medical units, sections, and individuals operate from planned, prescribed loads and from existing pre-positioned stockpiles.
- During initial deployment phase, each division support medical company (DSMC) and forward support medical company (FSMC) will receive a preconfigured medical resupply push-package every 48 hours from pre-positioned stock. These push-packages will continue until the Corps MEDLOG battalion is established.
- The battalion aid station (BAS) will receive resupply from the FSMC. This can be accomplished through direct requisition or through backhaul from ambulance runs.
- Individual combat medics will receive resupply from the ambulance crew or directly from the BAS.
- The Combat Lifesaver will receive resupply from the combat medic, the ambulance, or directly from the BAS.
- The individual soldier will receive his or her medical supplies directly from the BAS prior to deployment.

Medications for Individuals

o Individuals who require daily medications are required to bring a 6-month supply of their medications with them when deploying.

Set Up an Oxygen Tank

Performance Steps

1 Obtain the necessary equipment.

o Oxygen tank (cylinder); see **Figure 29**

> **note**
>
> Check the oxygen cylinder tag (**Figure 30**) to determine whether the tank is "Full," "In Use" (partially full), or "Empty."

CAUTION

Always ensure that the tank selected contains oxygen and not some other gas. U.S. oxygen tanks are color coded (painted) green. The international color code is white.

o Cylinder regulator with flowmeter (**Figure 31**)

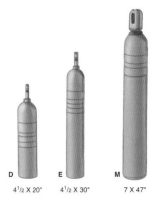

D   E   M
4¹/₂ X 20"   4¹/₂ X 30"   7 X 47"

Figure 29 Oxygen tanks.

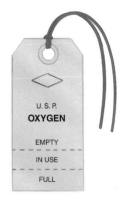

U.S.P.
OXYGEN

EMPTY

IN USE

FULL

Figure 30 Oxygen cylinder tag.

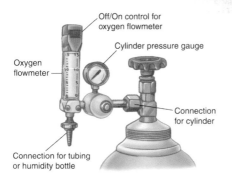

Figure 31 Cylinder regulator.

Off/On control for oxygen flowmeter

Cylinder pressure gauge

Oxygen flowmeter

Connection for cylinder

Connection for tubing or humidity bottle

note

(1) When the cylinder regulator pressure gauge reads 200 PSI or lower, the oxygen tank is considered empty. (2) The pressure-compensated flowmeter is affected by gravity and must be maintained in an upright position. The Bourdon gauge flowmeter is not affected by gravity and can be used in any position.

○ Humidifier
○ Sterile water
○ Nonsparking cylinder wrench
○ Oxygen tank transport carrier and/or stand
○ Oxygen delivery device ordered by the physician (nasal cannula or mask)
○ Warning signs
  ■ "NO SMOKING"
  ■ "OXYGEN IN USE"

CAUTION

Because of the extreme pressure in oxygen tanks, they should be handled with great care. Do not allow tanks to be banged together, dropped, or knocked over.

2 Secure the oxygen cylinder according to the following guidelines:

○ Upright position or in accordance with local SOP
○ Secured with straps or in a stand
○ Away from doors and areas of high traffic

3 Remove the cylinder valve cap.

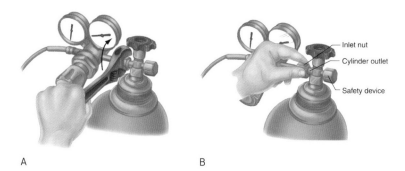

Figure 32 A: Tightening the inlet nut with a wrench. B: Tightening the inlet nut by hand.

> **note**
>
> The cylinder valve cap may be noisy or difficult to remove. However, the threads of the cylinder cap should never be oiled.

4 Use either the handwheel or a nonsparking wrench to "crack" (slowly open and quickly close) the cylinder to flush out any debris.

5 Attach the regulator to the cylinder.

O M cylinder
- Hold the gauge in an upright position.
- Insert the cylinder regulator inlet into the oxygen cylinder's threaded outlet in an upright position.
- Hand-tighten the inlet nut, located on the cylinder regulator, and then completely tighten the inlet nut with a nonsparking wrench (**Figure 32**).

6 Open the valve to test for leaks, and then close it.

> **note**
>
> If there is a leak, check the regulator connection and obtain a new regulator and/or tank, if necessary.

o D or E cylinder

- Locate the three holes on the oxygen cylinder stem and ensure that an O-ring is present. See **Figure 33**.

note

If the O-ring is not present, an oxygen leak will occur.

- Examine the yoke attachment and locate the three corresponding pegs on the yoke attachment. See **Figure 34**.
- Slide the yoke attachment over the cylinder stem, ensuring that the pegs are seated in the proper holes.
- Turn the vise-like screw on the side of the yoke attachment to secure it.
- Open the valve to test for leaks, and then close it.

note

(1) If there is a leak, check the regulator connection and obtain a new regulator and/or tank, if necessary. (2) When in-wall oxygen is available, the flowmeter will be attached to the oxygen outlet as follows: (a) Turn the flow-adjusting valve of the flowmeter to the OFF position. (b) Insert the flowmeter adapter into the opening outlet and press until a firm connection is made.

7 Fill the humidifier bottle to the level indicated (about two thirds full) with sterile water.

8 Attach the humidifier to the flowmeter.

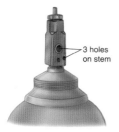

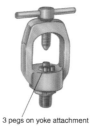

Figure 33 Attach yoke regulator stem.

Figure 34 Attach yoke regulator.

note

If an oxygen tube connector adapter is present, remove it from the flowmeter by turning the wing nut.

○ Attach the humidifier to the flowmeter with the wing nut on the humidifier.

note

Not all humidifiers have wing-style nuts. Some have regular bolt-style nuts.

○ Secure the nut by hand-tightening it.

note

Humidifiers and tubing should be changed at least once every 24 hours (or more often in accordance with local SOP).

9 Post warning signs.

CAUTION

"OXYGEN" and "NO SMOKING" signs should be posted in the areas where oxygen is in use or stored.

10 Report and/or record completion of the procedure.

Apply a Kendrick Extrication Device (KED)

Performance Steps

1 Identify the mechanism of injury that may be associated with spinal injuries.

○ Motor vehicle accidents
○ Head trauma

2 Apply the KED.

○ Manually stabilize the patient's head in a neutral in-line position.
○ Assess distal pulse, motor function, and sensation (PMS).
○ Apply the appropriate-sized cervical collar.
○ Position the immobilization device behind the patient.
○ Secure the device to the patient's torso.
○ Evaluate and pad behind the patient's head as necessary. Secure patient's head to device, using forehead and chin straps.
○ Evaluate and adjust the torso straps. They must be tight enough to prevent the device from moving up, down, and side to side excessively, but not so tight as to restrict the patient's breathing.
○ As needed, secure the patient's wrist and legs.
○ Reassess the patient's distal pulse, motor function, and sensation (PMS), and transfer the patient to a long spineboard.

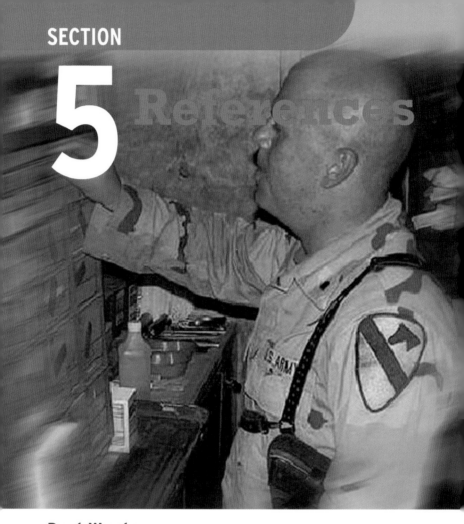

Root Words

Root Word	Meaning
aden	gland
angi	vessel
arthr	joint
bio	life
carcin	cancer
cephal	head
cerebr	brain
cerv	neck
chol	bile
chondr	cartilage
cost	rib

crani	skull
cyst	bladder
cyt	cell
derm	skin
electr	electricity
emesis	vomit
encephal	brain
enter	intestine
erythr	red
esthesia	feeling/sensation
febr	fever
gastr	stomach
gen	producing
glu/gly	sugar
gynec	woman
hema/hemat/hemo	blood
hepat	liver
hyster	uterus
laryng	larynx
lip	fat
lith	stone
mening	membrane
myel	marrow/spine
myo	muscle
nephr	kidney
ophthalm	eye
onc	tumor mass
osteo	bone
oto	ear
phleb	vein
pneum	lung/air
proct	rectum/anus
psych	soul/mind
pulm	lung
pyel	pelvis
pyo	pus
radi	ray
rhin	nose
scler	hard
scopy	examination
tendo	tendon
thromb	blood clot
toxin	poison
uro/uria	urine
vaso	vessel
veno	vein

Prefixes

Prefix	Meaning
a/an	absence of/without
ab	away from
ad	toward
ante	before/in front of
anti	against
bi	two/both/double
brady	slow
contra	opposite/against
cyano	blue
dys	difficulty
ec/ecto	outside
endo	within/inside
erythro	red
hemi	half
hyper	excessive/above/beyond
hypo	too little/low/below
inter	between
intra	inside
leuko	white
peri	around/surrounding
post	after
pre/pro	before/in front of
retro	backward/behind/in back of
semi	half
sub	under/beneath/below
super/supra	above/beyond/superior
tachy	fast

Suffixes

Suffix	Meaning
ac/al/ar/ic	pertaining to
algia	pain
cele	swelling/tumor
centesis	puncture
cis	cut
cyte	cell
ectasis	expansion/dilation
ectomy	removal/excision
emia	blood
genic	producing/originating
gram	record

iasis	condition/formation of/presence of
ist	one who specializes in
itis	inflammation
logy	process/study
lysis	breakdown/destruction
megaly	enlargement
oma	tumor
opsy	to view
osis	condition
otomy/tomy	cutting open
pathy	disease
sclerosis	hardening
scopy	examination/inspection

Common Medical Terms

Term	Meaning
afebrile	without fever
arteriosclerosis	hardening of the arteries
atherosclerosis	build-up, blockage, or narrowing of an artery
bradycardia	slow heart rate
bradypnea	slow breathing
bronchitis	inflammation of the bronchi
cardiovascular	pertaining to the heart and vessels
cyanosis	condition of blueness
dyspnea	difficulty breathing
endocarditis	inflammation within the heart
endotracheal	within the trachea
gastroenteritis	inflammation of the stomach and intestine
hematoma	blood-filled tumor
hematuria	blood in the urine
hepatitis	inflammation of the liver
hyperglycemia	high blood sugar
hypertension	high blood pressure
hypoglycemia	low blood sugar
hypotension	low blood pressure
intercostal	between the ribs
intracerebral	within the brain
intracranial	within the cranium
laryngoscopy	examination of the larynx with an instrument
myocardial	pertaining to the heart muscle
pathology	study of disease
splenectomy	removal of the spleen
tachycardia	rapid heart rate
tachypnea	faster than normal breathing
thyroidotomy	incision into the thyroid

Medical Abbreviations

Abbreviation	Meaning
ac	before meals
A/E	air evacuation
AD	right ear
A&D	admission and discharge
ADL	activities of daily living
ad lib	as desired
adm	admission; admit; admitted
afeb	afebrile; without fever
AMA	against medical advice
amb	ambulatory
ap	before dinner
A&P	anterior and posterior
APC	aspirin (acetylsalicylic acid), phenacetin, and caffeine
aq	water
AS	left ear
ASA	acetylsalicylic acid (aspirin)
ASAP	as soon as possible
AU	both ears
B/A	backache
BAT	blood alcohol test
BCP, OCP	birth control pills, oral contraceptive pills
bid, BID	twice a day
BM	bowel movement
BP	blood pressure
BRP	bathroom privileges
BS	bowel or breath sound(s)
BSA	body surface area
Bx	biopsy
C	centigrade
c̄	with
CA	cardiac arrest
Ca	calcium, cancer, carcinoma
cap	capsule
cath	catheter
CBC	complete blood count
CC	chief complaint
cc	cubic centimeter
CDC	Centers for Disease Control and Prevention
c/o	complaint of
CO	carbon monoxide
CO_2	carbon dioxide

CPR	cardiopulmonary resuscitation
CXR	chest x-ray
d/c	discontinue
D&C	dilatation and curettage
DJD	degenerative joint disease
DOA	dead on arrival
D5NS	5% dextrose in saline
D_5W	5% dextrose in water
Dx	diagnosis
EBL	estimated blood loss
ECG/EKG	electrocardiogram
E. coli	*Escherichia coli*
EMS	emergency medical services
ENT	ear, nose, throat
ER	emergency room
EtOH	ethyl alcohol
exam	examination
F	Fahrenheit
fb	foreign body
FBS	fasting blood sugar
FDA	Food and Drug Administration
ff	force fluids
fib	fibrillation
fx	fracture
g	grams
GI	gastrointestinal
gt; gtt	drop; drops
GU	genitourinary
GYN	gynecology
H	hydrogen
H_2O	water
HBP	high blood pressure
HEENT	head, eyes, ears, nose, throat
H&P	history and physical
HR	heart rate
hr	hour
hs	hour of sleep
Hx	history
IDDM	insulin-dependent diabetes mellitus
IM	intramuscular
I&O	intake and output
IO	intraosseous
IV	intravenous
K	potassium
kg	kilogram

continued

KUB	kidney, ureter, bladder
LOC	level of consciousness; loss of consciousness
LOS	length of stay
L	left
LP	lumbar puncture
L-S	lumbosacral
LUE	left upper extremity
mg	milligram
mL	milliliter
MVC	motor vehicle crash
N/C	no complaints
neg	negative
NKA, NKDA	no known allergies, no known drug allergies
nl	normal
nl BS	normal bowel sounds
NPO	nothing by mouth
ns, NS	normal saline
NSR	normal sinus rhythm
NTG	nitroglycerin
O_2	oxygen
OS	left eye
OD	right eye
OU	both eyes
OT	occupational therapy
PA	physician's assistant
P&A	percussion and auscultation
pc	after meals
PDR	*Physician's Desk Reference*
po, PO	by mouth
pos	positive
post-op	postoperative
pre-op	preoperative
prn, PRN	as needed
PT	physical therapy
pt	patient
PULHES	physical profile factors
PVC	premature ventricular contraction
qd	every day
qh	every hour
qhs	every evening
q2h, q3h, etc.	every 2 hours, every 3 hours, etc.
qid, QID	four times a day
QNS	quantity not sufficient
qod, QOD	every other day
R	right
Rx	prescription

RBC	red blood cells
rehab	rehabilitation
RN	registered nurse
R/O	rule out
ROM	range of motion
RR	recovery room
RTC	return to clinic
SC (see also SQ)	subcutaneous
SIW	self-inflicted wound
SOAP	progress note/charting format (subjective, objective, assessment, and plan)
SQ (see also SC)	subcutaneous
staph	staphyloccus
stat	immediately and once only
strep	streptococcus
sx	symptoms
S/S	signs and symptoms
T	temperature
tab	tablet
tid, TIB	three times a day
TPR	temperature, pulse, respirations
UA	urinalysis
UE	upper extremity
ULQ	upper left quadrant
URI	upper respiratory infection
URQ	upper right quadrant
UTI	urinary tract infection
VD	venereal disease
VO	verbal order
vs	vital signs
WBC	white blood count
WIA	wounded in action
wk	week
WNL	within normal limits
wt	weight
X	times
YOB	year of birth
ii	two
iii	three
iv	four
v	five

Medical Symbols

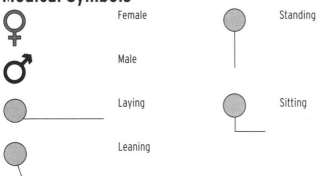

♀	Female
♂	Male
	Laying
	Leaning
	Standing
	Sitting

Vital Signs

Adult Vital Signs

Pulse	60 to 100 beats/min
Blood pressure	90 to 140 mm Hg (systolic) 60 to 90 mm Hg (diastolic)
Respirations	12 to 20 breaths/min

Pediatric Vital Signs

	Heart Rate (beats/min)		Blood Pressure (mm Hg)		
Age	Awake	Sleeping	Systolic	Diastolic	Respiratory Rate (breaths/min)
Neonate	100-180	80-160	70-100	50-65	30-60
6 months	120-160	80-180	87-105	53-66	25-50
2 years	80-150	70-120	90-106	55-67	18-35
5 years	80-110	60-90	94-109	56-69	17-27
10 years	70-110	60-90	102-117	62-75	15-23
>10 years	55-100	50-90	105-128	66-80	10-23

Labs

Blood Routine Tests

Test	Normal Values
Hemoglobin	Men: 13.5-17.5% Women: 11.5-16.5%
Total WBC count	Adults: 4,000-11,000/mm^3

Differential count	Neutrophils: 40-75%
	Eosinophils: 1-6%
	Lymphocytes: 10-45%
	Monocytes: 2-10%
	Basophils: 0-1%
ESR (Westergren), 1 hr	Men: 1-10 mm
	Women: 5-15 mm
Platelet count	150,000-400,000 mm^3
Reticulocyte count	Adults: 0.2-2.0%
RBC (erythrocyte) count	Men: 4.5-6.5 million/mm^3
	Women: 3.8-5.8 million/mm^3
Mean corpuscular volume	75-97 fL
Mean corpuscular hemoglobin	26-33 pg
Mean corpuscular hemoglobin concentration	32-35%
Hematocrit (PCV)	Men: 40-54%
	Women: 37-47%

ESR, erythrocyte sedimentation rate; PCV, packed cell volume; RBC, red blood cell; WBC, white blood cell.

Blood Special Tests

Test	Normal Values
Fasting blood sugar	20-120 mg/dL
Oxygen saturation	95-99%

Formulary

Antibiotics

Azithromycin (Zithromax; Z-PAK)

Description	• Antibiotic
Indications	• Mild to moderate susceptible infections, including acute bacterial sinusitis, acute otitis media, community-acquired pneumonia, pharyngitis/tonsillitis, uncomplicated bacterial skin infections, urethritis, cervicitis
Contraindications	• Known hypersensitivity to the drug
Precautions	• Avoid aluminum- or magnesium-containing antacids. • Pneumonia: Oral treatment is for mild, community-acquired cases suitable for outpatient therapy only. • Hypersensitivity reactions may recur after initial successful symptomatic treatment. • Adverse reactions: GI upset, abdominal pain, rash, chest pain.
Dosage/Route	• 500 mg once daily for 1 day, then 250 mg once daily for 4 days

Cefazolin Sodium (Ancef)

Description	• Cephalosporin C antibiotic that acts against gram-negative organisms
Indications	• Severe infections of the urinary and biliary tracts, skin, soft tissue, and bone; open heart surgery; endocarditis
Contraindications	• Hypersensitivity to any cephalosporin and related antibiotics
Precautions	• History of penicillin sensitivity, impaired renal function, and patients on sodium restriction
Dosage/Route	• Moderate to severe infections: Adult, IV/IM: 250 mg to 2 g every 8 hours, up to 2 g every 4 hours (maximum 12 g daily) • Surgical prophylaxis: Adult, IV/IM: 1-2 g 30 to 60 minutes before surgery, then every 8 hours for 24 hours

Cefotetan

Description	• Antibiotic
Indications	• Prophylactic use in unconscious patients who have received a battlefield wound
Contraindications	• Known hypersensitivity to the drug
Precautions	• Cefotetan is a cephalosporin antibiotic, which has a cross-sensitivity reaction to penicillin (i.e., if people are allergic to penicillin, there is a possibility that they will be allergic to cephalosporins). Identify soldiers who are allergic to penicillin prior to deployment and have substitute antibiotics for these soldiers. • Abdominal pain and diarrhea may occur.
Dosage/Route	• 2 g IV push over 3 to 5 minutes, which may be repeated at 12-hour intervals until evacuation

Cephalexin (Keflex)

Description	• Antibiotic
Indications	• Susceptible infections, including otitis media, skin and skin structures, bone, and respiratory or genitourinary tract
Contraindications	• Known hypersensitivity to the drug
Precautions	• Cross-reactivity for those with penicillin allergy • Adverse reactions: GI upset, diarrhea, headache, fatigue, dizziness, hypersensitivity reactions, itch
Dosage/Route	• 250-500 mg every 6 hours for 7 to 10 days

Ceftriaxone Sodium (Rocephin)

Description	• Broad-spectrum antibiotic, cephalosporin (third generation). Stops bacterial cell wall synthesis, which renders cell walls osmotically unstable and leads to cell death.

Indications	• Gram-negative organisms; gram-positive organisms; lower, serious respiratory tract infections; urinary tract infections; skin, bone, and joint infections; gonococcal infections; intra-abdominal infections; septicemia; and meningitis (bacterial)
Contraindications	• Hypersensitivity to cephalosporins; infants younger than 1 year
Precautions	• Nursing mothers
Dosage/Route	• Adult, IV/IM: 1-2 g every day or in two equal doses • Uncomplicated gonorrhea: 260 mg IM as a single dose • Meningitis: Adult, IM/IV: 100 mg/kg per day in equal doses every 12 hours

Ciprofloxacin (Cipro)

Description	• Antibiotic
Indications	• Susceptible infections, including lower respiratory tract, skin and skin structures, bone and joint, acute sinusitis, UTI, bacterial prostatitis, infectious diarrhea, and uncomplicated urethral and cervical gonorrhea; anthrax exposure
Contraindications	• Known hypersensitivity to the drug
Precautions	• GI upset, headache, convulsions, dizziness, nervousness, insomnia, nightmares, paranoia, rash, photosensitivity, Stevens-Johnson syndrome, myalgia • Increases theophylline levels • Potentiates caffeine
Dosage/Route	• 500 mg twice daily for 10 days

Doxycycline

Description	• Antibiotic
Indications	• Is effective for selected infections of the upper respiratory tract or of the genitourinary tract; malaria prophylaxis
Contraindications	• Pregnant women: Causes disturbances in the development of the teeth and bones of the fetus

Precautions	• Adverse reactions
	  ■ Approximately 3% to 4% of the treated subjects complain about nausea.
	  ■ Abdominal pains and diarrhea are less common.
	  ■ Doxycycline can cause a cutaneous photosensitivity: Inform patient of increased risk of sunburn and sensitivity to sun; advise patient to wear sunscreen.
	• Interactions
	  ■ Concomitant administration of antacids causes a reduced absorption of the antibiotic.

Dosage/Route	• 100 mg once daily to twice daily. Duration varies depending on indication. • Malaria prophylaxis: 100 mg daily; begin 1 to 2 weeks before, continue during and 4 weeks after travel to malarious area.

Gatifloxacin

Description	• Antibiotic
Indications	• Part of combat pill pack to be taken by soldiers who have received a battlefield wound
Contraindications	• Previous anaphylactic reaction to penicillin or cephalosporins
Precautions	• Adverse effects: Urticaria, allergic reactions. Identify soldiers who are allergic to penicillin prior to deployment and have substitute antibiotics for these soldiers. • Dizziness, nervousness, agitation, paranoia, insomnia, palpitations, changes in blood sugar. • Abdominal pain and diarrhea may occur.
Dosage/Route	• 400 mg orally once a day for 7 to 10 days

Antifungals

Clotrimazole Cream (Lotrimin)

Description	• Antifungal
Indications	• Used to treat tinea pedis (athlete's foot), tinea cruris, and tinea corporis
Contraindications	• Patients with known hypersensitivity to the drug or its components

Precautions	• Side effects: Stinging; erythema; edema vesication; pruritus and urticaria
	• Considerations
	  ■ Apply to dry skin.
	  ■ Cleanse skin thoroughly before applying the medication.
	  ■ Signs of clinical improvement should be anticipated within 1 week of use. Report signs of condition worsening, skin irritation, or no improvement after 4 weeks of therapy.

Dosage/Route	• Apply small amount to affected area twice a day, morning and night, or as directed by the physician.

Diflucan

Description	• Antifungal
Indications	• Used to treat vaginal, oropharyngeal, and esophageal candidiasis
Contraindications	• Contraindicated in patients with known hypersensitivity to the drug
Precautions	• Monitor liver function. Discontinue if liver disease or progressively worsening rash develops.
Dosage/Route	• Varies widely, depending on indication. 150 mg for one dose.

Miconazole 2% Cream

Description	• Antifungal
Indications	• Used to treat tinea pedis (athlete's foot), tinea cruris, and tinea corporis
Contraindications	• Contraindicated in patients with known hypersensitivity to the drug
Precautions	• Side effects: Skin irritation; burning; maceration; allergic contact dermatitis
Dosage/Route	• Apply sparingly twice a day to the affected area for 2 to 4 weeks.

Tolnaftate (Tinactin)

Description	• Antifungal
Indications	• Superficial fungal infections of the skin: tinea pedis, tinea cruris, tinea corporis, tinea versicolor
Contraindications	• Patients hypersensitive to the drug or its active ingredients
Precautions	• No significant precautions
Dosage/Route	• Apply to affected area twice daily for 2 to 6 weeks.

Antihistamines

Cetirizine (Zyrtec)

Description	• Antihistamine
Indications	• Seasonal allergic rhinitis, perennial allergic rhinitis, chronic urticaria
Contraindications	• Known hypersensitivity to the drug
Precautions	• Avoid aluminum- or magnesium-containing antacids. • Adverse reactions: GI upset, headache, back pain, viral infection, sinusitis, dizziness, drowsiness.
Dosage/Route	• 10 mg orally once daily

Chlorpheniramine Maleate (Chlor-Trimeton)

Description	• Antihistamine
Indications	• Symptomatic relief of rhinitis and seasonal allergy symptoms
Contraindications	• Hypersensitivity to antihistamines • Lower respiratory tract symptoms • Narrow-angle glaucoma • Severe hypertension • Severe cardiovascular disease • Bronchial asthma • Patients taking MAO inhibitors

Precautions	• Side effects: Low incidence of side effects
	  ▪ Drowsiness
	  ▪ Dizziness
	  ▪ Dryness of mouth and nose

- Considerations
  - Drug may cause drowsiness.
  - Driving and other potentially hazardous activities should be avoided until the response to the drug is known.
  - Avoid alcohol use when taking this drug. Antihistamines have additive effects with alcohol.

Dosage/Route
- 8 mg orally every 8 hours (three times daily)
- Maximum daily (24 hours) dose: 24 mg

Dimenhydrinate (Dramamine)

Description	• Produces temporary relief of various allergic reactions by blocking histamine secretions
Indications	• Prevention and treatment of motion sickness
Contraindications	• Known hypersensitivity to drug or its components
Precautions	• Adverse reactions ■ Central nervous system: Drowsiness, dizziness, headache, confusion, vertigo ■ Cardiovascular: Palpitations, hypotension, tachycardia ■ EENT: Blurred vision, dry respiratory passages ■ Gastrointestinal: Dry mouth, nausea, vomiting, diarrhea, anorexia ■ Respiratory: Wheezing, thickened bronchial secretions ■ Skin: Photosensitivity, urticaria, rash ■ Other: Anaphylaxis, tightness of the chest
Dosage/Route	• 50-100 mg orally every 4 to 6 hours. For prevention, take 30 minutes before motion exposure.

Diphenhydramine Hydrochloride (Benadryl)

Description	• Produces temporary relief of various allergic reactions by blocking histamine secretions
Indications	• Allergic reactions (urticaria), motion sickness, vertigo, reactions to blood or plasma, and anaphylaxis as an adjunct to epinephrine and other standard measures after acute symptoms have been controlled
Contraindications	• Hypersensitivity to antihistamines, lower respiratory tract symptoms (including acute asthma), narrow-angle glaucoma, gastrointestinal obstruction, and bladder neck obstructions
Precautions	• History of asthma, convulsive disorders, increased intraocular pressure, hyperthyroidism, cardiovascular disease, diabetes mellitus
Dosage/Route	• Allergic symptoms, adult: 25-50 mg orally three or four times a day (maximum 300 mg daily) • IV/IM: 10-50 mg every 4 to 6 hours (maximum 400 mg daily) • Nonproductive cough, adult: 25 mg every 4 to 6 hours (maximum 100 mg daily)

Fexofenadine (Allegra)

Description	• Antihistamine
Indications	• Allergic rhinitis
Contraindications	• Known hypersensitivity to the drug
Precautions	• Avoid aluminum- or magnesium-containing antacids. • Adverse reactions: Somnolence, fatigue, dry mouth, pharyngitis, dizziness, drowsiness.
Dosage/Route	• 180 mg once daily or 60 mg twice daily

Antimalarials

Mefloquine

Description	• Antimalarial
Indications	• Prophylaxis of *Plasmodium falciparum* (including chloroquine-resistant strains) and *Plasmodium vivax* malaria; treatment of mild to moderate acute malaria due to susceptible strains of *P. falciparum* or *P. vivax*
Contraindications	• Quinine, quinidine, or related allergy
Precautions	• Discontinue prophylactic therapy if central nervous system disturbances occur. Take with food and 8 oz water.
Dosage/Route	• Prophylaxis: 250 mg once weekly starting 1 week before departure, continuing during travel to endemic areas and for 4 weeks after return

Primaquine

Description	• Antimalarial
Indications	• Used for the treatment of *P. vivax* or *P. ovale* malaria to provide a radical cure after a clinical attack has been confirmed by blood smear or serologic titer to be caused by one of these plasmodial species. Because primaquine is not generally active against asexual erythrocytic forms of plasmodia, a blood schizonticidal agent (preferably chloroquine) is always given in conjunction with primaquine for the treatment of *P. ovale* or *P. vivax* malaria. • Primaquine also is used in conjunction with chloroquine or another suitable antimalarial agent to decrease the risk of delayed primary attacks and relapse of *P. ovale* and *P. vivax* malaria. The U.S. Centers for Disease Control and Prevention (CDC) currently states that prophylaxis with primaquine is indicated only for returning travelers (terminal prophylaxis) when exposure to malaria occurred in areas where *P. ovale* and *P. vivax* are endemic.
Contraindications	• Retinal or visual field changes
Precautions	• Use with caution in patients with hepatic disease or alcoholism or in conjunction with known hepatotoxic drugs.
Dosage/Route	• 30 mg per day (two tablets daily) has been shown to provide excellent protection against *P. falciparum* and *P. vivax* malaria in Indonesia, Kenya, and Colombia.

Cardiac Medications

Nitroglycerin (Nitrostat)

Description	• It was originally believed that nitrates dilate the coronary blood vessels, thereby increasing blood flow to the heart. It is now believed that atherosclerosis limits coronary dilation and that the benefits of nitrates are due to the dilation of arterioles and veins in the periphery. The result is a reduction in the preload, and to a lesser extent in the afterload, which decreases the workload of the heart and lowers myocardial oxygen demand. Nitroglycerin is lipid soluble and is thought to enter the body from the GI tract through the lymphatics, rather than portal blood.
Indications	• Angina pectoris; ischemic chest pain; hypertension; and congestive heart failure (CHF) associated with acute myocardial infarction
Contraindications	• Hypersensitivity, hypotension, head injury, cerebral hemorrhage, uncorrected hypovolemia, constrictive pericarditis, pericardial tamponade
Precautions	• Increased susceptibility to hypotension in the elderly. • Use in pregnancy is safe. • Nitroglycerin decomposes in light and heat. Must be kept in airtight containers. • Oral medication. Sublingual use will produce a stinging sensation. If given IV, use an infusion pump for precise flow rate. • When applied use body substance isolation (BSI); the user of the medication may experience syncope.
Dosage/Route	• Adult: 0.3 to 0.4 tablet sublingually; may be repeated at 5-minute intervals two times. • Metered spray: Spray onto oral mucosa using a lingual aerosol canister that delivers 0.4 mg/min; may be repeated at 5-minute intervals two times. • Infusion: 200-400 (mg/mL at a rate of 10-20 (mg/min; increase by 5-10 (mg/min every 5 to 10 minutes until desired effect is achieved.

Gastrointestinal Medications

Calcium Carbonate Tablets

Description	• Antacids
Indications	• Relief of transient symptoms of hyperacidity, such as in acid indigestion and heartburn • Calcium supplement
Contraindications	• Patients with hypercalcemia and hypercalciuria. • Do not use in patients with calcium loss due to immobilization, severe renal disease, or renal calculi; GI hemorrhage or obstruction; or cardiac disease.

Precautions	• Side effects
	■ Constipation or laxative effect
	■ Acid rebound
	■ Nausea
	■ Flatulence
	• Considerations
	■ When used as an antacid, take 1 hour after meals and at bedtime.
	■ Acid rebound, which generally occurs after repeated use of antacids for 1 or 2 weeks, can lead to chronic use.
	■ Caution patient not to use antacids for more than 2 weeks without medical supervision.
Dosage/Route	• Antacid: 0.5–2.0 g orally 4 to 6 times per day
	• Calcium supplement: 1–2 g orally every 8 or every 12 hours

Hemorrhoidal Supositories

Description	• Prompt relief for the itching and pain associated with hemorrhoids
Indications	• Hemorrhoids, anorectal inflammation, pruritus ani
Contraindications	• None
Precautions	• Side effects: Localized irritation in the rectal area
Dosage/Route	• 1 rectally 2 to 3 times daily

Kaolin Mixture with Pectin (Kaopectate)

Description	• White powdered substance. The container must be shaken to mix the ingredients.
Indications	• Antidiarrheal
Contraindications	• Patient is constipated or dehydrated
Precautions	• Ensure that the patient drinks a lot of water when on this medication.
Dosage/Route	• Adult: 4 to 8 tablespoons (60–120 mL) after each loose bowel movement

Loperamide (Imodium)

Description	• Antidiarrhetic
Indications	• Acute nonspecific diarrhea
Contraindications	• None
Precautions	• Side effects: Constipation
Dosage/Route	• 4 mg, then 2 mg after each loose stool; maximum 16 mg per day

Pepto-Bismol

Description	• Antimicrobial
Indications	• Diarrhea
Contraindications	• Varicella or influenza in children and teenagers

| **Precautions** | • Adverse reactions: Darkened tongue and/or stool |
| **Dosage/Route** | • 2 caplets or 30 mL every 30 to 60 minutes if needed; maximum 8 doses per day |

Promethazine (Phenergan)

Description	• Antiemetic
Indications	• Motion sickness, refractory nausea and vomiting. Used to combat morphine's side effect of nausea and vomiting.
Contraindications	• None
Precautions	• Sedation, disorientation, and dizziness. Do not use in ambulatory patients.
Dosage/Route	• IM or IV push dose of Phenergan is 25 or 50 mg. • If the dose is given intramuscularly, inject the medication deep into a large muscle mass. • If the drug is given IV, a *slow* IV push should be given over 1 to 2 minutes. Dilute the medication with several cubic centimeters of normal saline.

Simethicone (Mylanta Gas)

Description	• Either liquid or tablet form. Decreases gas production, coalesces gas bubbles, and facilitates the passage of gas through belching and expelling flatus. Antacids increase the gastric pH, thereby neutralizing gastric acidity. Composed of inorganic salts of aluminum, magnesium, calcium, or sodium.
Indications	• Antiflatulent, antacid
Contraindications	• Massive gastrointestinal bleeds
Precautions	• Renal insufficiency
Dosage/Route	• Adult: 5-15 mL orally four times daily, or 40-125 mg tablet four times daily with meals

Headache Medications

Acetaminophen (Tylenol)

Description	• Produces analgesia; reduces fever by direct action on the hypothalamus heat-regulating center, which causes peripheral vasodilatation, sweating, and dissipation of heat.
Indications	• Analgesic; antipyretic substitute for aspirin if aspirin is not tolerated
Contraindications	• Drug is hepatotoxic (overdose treatment is oral acetylcysteine [Mucomyst]); hypersensitivity to acetaminophen.
Precautions	• Anemic patients, alcoholism, malnutrition, thrombocytopenia
Dosage/Route	• Adult: 1 to 2 tablets (325-650 mg) orally every 4 to 6 hours; maximum 4 g daily

Acetylsalicylic Acid (ASA)/Aspirin

Description	• Stops the formation of prostaglandins involved in the production of inflammation, pain, and fever responses
Indications	• Antipyretic, anti-inflammatory, and analgesic
Contraindications	• Hypersensitivity to ASA, increased bleeding time; toxicity manifests with tinnitus and hearing loss. Do not use in teens and children due to the possible link to Reye's syndrome. Prolonged bleeding, GI ulcers, bleeding or other problems, petechiae, easy bruising, hemolytic anemia, thrombocytopenia, dizziness, confusion, drowsiness. Urticaria, anaphylactic shock. Chronic rhinitis, vitamin K deficiencies.
Precautions	• Do not use with otic diseases, in children with fever and dehydration, or in patients with cardiac disease or hepatic impairment. Soldiers should avoid aspirin and other nonsteroidal anti-inflammatory medicines while in a combat zone because of their detrimental effects on hemostasis.
Dosage/Route	• Adult: 1 to 2 tablets (325–650 mg) orally every 4 hours; maximum 4 g daily

Midrin (Acetaminophen, Isometheptene, and Dichloralphenazone)

Description	• Sympathomimetic plus sedative plus analgesic
Indications	• Tension and vascular headache, migraine
Contraindications	• Glaucoma; severe renal, cardiac, hypertensive, or hepatic disease
Precautions	• Peripheral vascular disease, recent myocardial infarction, gastritis, hypertension • Adverse reactions: Dizziness, drowsiness, sympathomimetic effects, rash
Dosage/Route	• Tension: 1 to 2 capsules every 4 hours; maximum 8 capsules per day • Migraine: 2 capsules once, then 1 capsule every 1 hour; maximum 5 capsules per 12 hours

Sumatriptan Succinate (Imitrex)

Description	• 5HT1 receptor agonist that causes vasoconstriction
Indications	• Acute treatment of migraine or cluster headaches
Contraindications	• Known hypersensitivity to the drug, uncontrolled hypertension, ischemic heart disease
Precautions	• Adverse reactions: Tingling, hot sensation; flushing; chest, neck, jaw discomfort; dizziness; muscle pain or weakness; fatigue, drowsiness; headache; anxiety; sweating; seizures
Dosage/Route	• Oral: 25–100 mg once followed by second dose in 2 hours

- Nasal spray: 5-20 mg intranasally once, repeat after 2 hours; maximum 40 mg per day
- Subcutaneous injection: 6 mg; up to two injections, with at least 1 hour between injections

Hypoglycemic Agents

Dextrose 50%/D50W

Description	• The term *dextrose* is used to describe the six-carbon sugar D-glucose, the principle form of carbohydrate utilized by the body. D50 is used in emergency care to treat hypoglycemia, and in the management of coma of unknown etiology. Carbohydrate, hypertonic solution.
Indications	• Hypoglycemia, altered level of consciousness, coma of unknown etiology, refractory cardiac arrest
Contraindications	• Intracranial pressure, intracranial hemorrhages, known or suspected cerebrovascular accident (CVA) in the absence of hypoglycemia
Precautions	• Draw blood sample prior to administration if possible. Perform dextrose stick prior to administration if possible. Extravasation may cause tissue necrosis; use a large vein and aspirate occasionally to ensure route patency. D50 may sometimes precipitate severe neurologic symptoms in thiamin-deficient patients (e.g., alcoholics).
Dosage/Route	• Adult: 12.5-25.0 g slowly IV; may be repeated once.

Muscle Relaxants

Cyclobenzaprine (Flexeril)

Description	• Muscle relaxant
Indications	• Short-term treatment of muscle spasm
Contraindication	• Patients hypersensitive to the drug
Precautions	• Adverse reactions ■ Central nervous system: Drowsiness, dizziness, headache, insomnia, fatigue, nervousness, confusion ■ Cardiovascular: Tachycardia, arrhythmias, palpitations, hypotension, vasodilation ■ EENT: Blurred vision ■ Gastrointestinal: Nausea, dyspepsia, abnormal taste, constipation, dry mouth
Dosage/Route	• 10 mg orally three times a day for 2 to 3 weeks

Diazepam (Valium)

Description	• Frequently used medication for anxiety and stress. In emergency care, it is used to treat alcoholic withdrawal and grand mal seizures. It acts upon the limbic, thalamic, and hypothalamic regions of the central nervous system to induce calming effects. Sedative; anticonvulsant.

Indications	· Used widely as an anticonvulsant; it is actually a weak anticonvulsant and has short duration time.
	· Nerve agent poisoning; acute anxiety attacks; alcohol withdrawal; muscle relaxant; seizure activity; and premedication for countershock or transcutaneous pacing (TCP).
Contraindications	· Hypersensitivity to the drug, substance abuse, coma, shock, and central nervous system depression as a result of a head injury.
Precautions	· Rapid IV administration may be followed by respiratory depression.
	· Vein irritation.
	· Short duration for anticonvulsant effect.
	· Reduce dose by 50% in elderly patients.
	· Resuscitation equipment should be ready.
Dosage/Route	· Seizure activity, adult: 5 mg over 2 minutes (up to 10 mg for most adults) IV every 10 to 15 minutes as needed (maximum dose 30 mg daily)
	· Anxiety, muscle spasm, convulsions, and alcohol withdrawal, adult: 2-10 mg orally twice daily to four times daily or 15-3 mg per day in sustained-release form
	· IV/IM: 2-10 mg; repeat if necessary in 3 to 4 hours

Methocarbamol (Robaxin)

Description	· Muscle relaxant
Indications	· As an adjunct in acute, painful musculoskeletal conditions
Contraindications	· Patients hypersensitive to the drug
Precautions	· Adverse reactions
	▪ Central nervous system: Drowsiness, dizziness, headache, light-headedness
	▪ Cardiovascular: Hypotension, bradycardia with IM or IV route
	▪ EENT: Blurred vision, conjunctivitis, nystagmus, diplopia
	▪ Gastrointestinal: Nausea, GI upset, metallic taste
Dosage/Route	· 1.5 g orally four times daily for 2 to 3 days, then 4 g daily in divided doses

Nerve Agent Antidote

Atropine Sulfate/Atropine

Description	· Blocks vagal impulses to the heart, which decreases atrioventricular conduction, increases heart rate, and increases cardiac output. Antisecretory action suppresses sweating, lacrimation, salivation, and secretions from the nose, mouth, pharynx, and bronchi. Produces mydriasis (dilation of pupils) and cycloplegia (paralysis of accommodation) by blocking the iris sphincter muscle and ciliary muscle.

Indications	• Treatment of nerve agent exposure, cardiac arrhythmias (heart blocks, bradycardia, arrest). Preoperatively to decrease oral and gastric secretions. Ophthalmic to dilate eyes. Oral inhalation for short treatment and prevention of bronchospasms associated with asthma, bronchitis, and chronic obstructive pulmonary disease (COPD), and as a drying agent for upper respiratory infections.
Contraindications	• Acute hemorrhage, hypersensitivity to belladonna alkaloids, bladder neck obstruction, diseases of the GI tract, severe ulcerative colitis, tachycardia secondary to cardiac insufficiency
Precautions	• Myocardial infarction, hypertension, hypotension, coronary artery disease, congestive heart failure, tachyarrhythmias, gastric ulcers, gastrointestinal infections, hyperthyroidism, chronic lung disease, hepatic or renal disease. May cause heat injuries in hot, dry climates.
Dosage/Route	• Nerve agent: Auto-injectors of 2 mg for IM use • Preoperative: 0.4-0.6 mg IM • Cardiac: 0.5-1.0 mg IV push (maximum 2 mg) • Ophthalmic: 1 drop of 1% solution

2-Pyridine Aldoxime Methochloride/Pralidoxime Chloride

Description	• An oxime. Oximes attach to the nerve agent that is stopping the cholinesterase secretions and break the agent-enzyme bond to restore the normal activity of the enzyme. Abnormal activity in skeletal muscle decreases, and normal strength returns.
Indications	• Nerve agent poisoning
Contraindications	• None noted
Precautions	• Could cause heat injury if used in a dry, hot environment.
Dosage/Route	• Adult: Give with the atropine auto-injector (Mark I kit), up to three sets depending on exposure to the nerve agent. If three sets of the Mark I kit are given, then give 10 mg Valium IM.

Pain Medications

Ibuprofen (Motrin)

Description	• Nonsteroidal anti-inflammatory drug (NSAID)
Indications	• Mild to moderate pain relief to include headaches (analgesia) and fever reduction (antipyretic)
Contraindications	• Patients with hypersensitivity to the drug • Patients with known ulcer disease

Precautions	• Side effects: Increases bleeding time for 8 hours
	  ▪ Gastrointestinal pain
	  ▪ Nausea
	  ▪ Occult gastrointestinal bleeding

- Considerations
  - Take with meals or milk to reduce GI side effects.
  - Do not use with aspirin or alcohol, which may increase risk of GI reactions.
  - Serious GI bleeding can occur in patients taking NSAIDs despite absence of symptoms.
  - Patients should be taught the signs and symptoms of GI bleeding (dark, tarry stools; coffee-ground stools; or bloody emesis) and instructed to notify the MD or PA immediately if they occur.

Dosage/Route	• For mild to moderate pain, 400-800 mg orally every 6 to 8 hours • For fever, 200-800 mg orally every 6 to 8 hours • Maximum daily dose (24 hours): 3,200 mg

Ketorolac (Toradol) IV/IM

Description	• Nonsteroidal anti-inflammatory drug
Indications	• Management of moderately severe, acute pain requiring opioid-level analgesia
Contraindications	• Aspirin allergy, peptic ulcer, gastrointestinal bleed or perforation, advanced renal impairment

Precautions	• Adverse reactions
	  ▪ Headache
	  ▪ Gastrointestinal pain/fullness, dyspepsia

Dosage/Route	• 30 mg IM or IV every 6 hours

Morphine Sulfate

Description	• A natural opium alkaloid used as a narcotic, an analgesic, and for sedation
Indications	• Severe acute or chronic pain; relieve dyspnea of acute left ventricular failure; pulmonary edema; and pain of a myocardial infarction
Contraindications	• Hypersensitivity to opiates; increased intracranial pressure; convulsive disorders; bronchial asthma and respiratory depression; diarrhea caused by poisoning until the toxic material has been eliminated
Precautions	• Oral solution: Dilute in approximately 30 mL or more of fluid or semisolid food. Extended-release tablet should not be broken in half, crushed, or chewed. • IV administration: Give direct. Dilute in 5 mL sterile water for injection. Store at 15-30°C (59-86°F). Avoid freezing. Protect all formulas from light.
Dosage/Route	• Adult, oral: 10-30 mg every 4 hours; extended-release tablet: 15-30 mg every 8 hours • IV: 2.5-15.0 mg every 4 hours • SC/IM: 5-20 mg every 4 hours • Rectal: 10-20 mg every 4 hours

Oxycodone and Acetaminophen (Percocet)

Description	• Opioid analgesic
Indications	• Moderate to moderately severe pain
Contraindications	• Known hypersensitivity to opiates
Precautions	• Head injury, increased intracranial pressure; acute abdominal conditions • Interactions: Potentiation with alcohol, other central nervous system depressants, MAO inhibitors, tricyclic antidepressants, anticholinergics
Dosage/Route	• 1 tablet every 6 hours as needed

Pulmonary Medications

Albuterol (Proventil)

Description	• Dilates the smooth muscles of the bronchi and uterus, and the vascular supply to the skeletal muscles. Produces bronchodilation regardless of route of administration, by relaxing the smooth muscles of the bronchial tree. This decreases airway resistance, facilitates mucus drainage, and increases vital capacity.
Indications	• To relieve bronchospasms associated with acute or chronic asthma, bronchitis, or other reversible obstructive airway disease
Contraindications	• Nursing mothers, and children younger than 2 years
Precautions	• Cardiovascular disease, hypertension, hyperthyroidism, diabetes mellitus, hypersensitivity to sympathomimetic amines or to fluorocarbon propellants used in inhalation aerosols
Dosage/Route	• Adult, oral: 2-4 mg three to four times per day. 4-8 mg of sustained-release form twice a day. • Inhaled: 1 to 2 inhalations every 4 to 6 hours.

Epinephrine 1:1000 (1 mg/1 cc)

Description	• Bronchodilator
Indications	• Used for bronchospasm, hypersensitivity (allergic) reactions, and anaphylaxis
Contraindications	• Patients with known hypersensitivity to the drug • Patients with narrow-angle glaucoma; hemorrhagic, traumatic, or cardiogenic shock; cardiac arrhythmias; or coronary insufficiency

Precautions	• Side effects
	  ▪ Nervousness
	  ▪ Restlessness
	  ▪ Palpitations
	  ▪ Tremors
	  ▪ Fear
	  ▪ Anxiety

- Headache
- Hypertension
- Nausea and vomiting
- Considerations
  - Drug of choice for acute anaphylactic reactions.
  - Patients allergic to insect stings should be taught to self-administer epinephrine.
  - Closely monitor vital signs after administration of the drug.

Dosage/Route	• 0.1–0.5 cc subcutaneously every 15 minutes as needed to treat acute symptoms

Reversal Agents

Naloxone Hydrochloride (Narcan)

Description	• Naloxone is a competitive narcotic antagonist that is used in the management and reversal of overdoses caused by narcotics and synthetic narcotics. Unlike other narcotic antagonists, which do not stop the analgesic properties of opiates, naloxone antagonizes *all* the actions of morphine and other opiates, including the analgesic properties.
Indications	• For the complete or partial reversal of central nervous system and respiratory depression induced by opioids • Decreased level of consciousness; coma of unknown origin • Narcotic agonist: Morphine sulfate, heroin, hydromorphone (Dilaudid), methadone, meperidine (Demerol), paregoric, fentanyl citrate (Sublimaze), oxycodone (Percodan), codeine, and propoxyphene (Darvon) • Narcotic agonist/antagonist: Butorphanol tartrate (Stadol), pentazocine (Talwin), and nalbuphine (Nubain)
Contraindications	• Hypersensitivity to Narcan • Respiratory depression not due to opiates
Precautions	• May precipitate withdrawal symptoms in narcotic-dependent patients (including neonates of narcotic-dependent mothers), with hypertension, tachycardia, and violent behavior.
Dosage/Route	• Adult: Begin with 2 mg IV, IM, SQ (or endotracheal diluted); may be repeated at 5-minute intervals to a maximum of 10 mg • Infusion: Mix 8 mg in 1,000 mL of D_5W; infuse at 0.8 mg/hr (100 mL/hr) titrated to desired effect.

Topical Medications

Analgesic Balm (Ben-Gay)

Description	• Topical analgesic
Indications	• Effective for relief of minor muscle aches
Contraindications	• None

Precautions	• Side effects: Possible rash
Dosage/Route	• Apply to affected area every 3 to 4 hours as needed.

Bacitracin

Description	• Anti-infective, antibiotic
Indications	• Topical for the treatment of superficial infections of the skin or eye
Contraindications	• Toxic reaction or renal dysfunction associated with bacitracin-impaired renal function
Precautions	• Myasthenia gravis, other neurological diseases; hypersensitivity to neomycin
Dosage/Route	• Adult: Apply thin layer to affected area twice or thrice daily. • Ophthalmic ointment: Apply in the conjunctiva sac 1 or more times per day.

Burrow's Solution/Domeboro Tablets

Description	• Astringent
Indications	• Solution prepared from either powder or tablets used as a soothing wet dressing to relieve inflammation of the skin resulting from insect bites, poison ivy, swelling, and athlete's foot
Contraindications	• None
Precautions	• Side effects: Localized rash. • Special instructions: Patient should be instructed to keep solution away from the eyes. Once in liquid form, Burrow's solution should be kept at room temperature for no more than 7 days.
Dosage/Route	• Dissolve one to two packets or tablets in 1 pint of water. Apply as wet dressing for four treatments of 30 minutes each daily.

Calamine Lotion

Description	• Drying agent
Indications	• Dries the oozing and weeping of poison ivy, poison oak, and poison sumac. Soothes the irritation of the most common skin rashes.
Contraindications	• None
Precautions	• None
Dosage/Route	• Apply to affected area as needed.

Chapstick

Description	• A stick of solidified petroleum jelly
Indications	• Very effective in providing relief for dry, chapped, or cracked lips
Contraindications	• None

Precautions	• None
Dosage/Route	• Apply to lips as needed.

Eugenol

Description	• Liquid substance used as a temporary filling for teeth and local analgesia
Indications	• Temporary dental filling
Contraindications	• Liver disease, skin disorders, and any eye diseases
Precautions	• Store in cool, dry areas in closed containers. Darkens and thickens upon exposure.
Dosage/Route	• Adult: Place a small layer on affected tooth, or teeth, as needed.

Foot Powder (with Undecylenic Acid)

Description	• Antifungal powder
Indications	• Effective against fungal infections of the foot, especially between the toes
Contraindications	• None
Precautions	• None
Dosage/Route	• Apply a light dusting to feet two to three times daily as needed.

Hydrocortisone 1% Cream

Description	• Topical anti-inflammatory
Indications	• For relief of inflammation and pruritus associated with contact dermatitis
Contraindications	• Patients with known hypersensitivity to the drug or its components
Precautions	• Side effects ■ Maceration of the skin ■ Secondary infection • Considerations ■ Gently wash skin before applying ointment. ■ Avoid applying near eyes or mucous membranes. ■ May be safely used on the face, groin, armpits, and under the breasts.
Dosage/Route	• Apply ointment to affected area sparingly daily one to four times a day until the acute phase is controlled, then reduce dosage to one to three times weekly, as needed.

Lindane (Kwell)

Description	• Topical anti-parasite drug
Indications	• Parasitic infestation (scabies, pediculosis)
Contraindications	• Patients with known hypersensitivity to the drug or its components
Precautions	• Adverse reactions: Dizziness, seizures, skin irritation

| **Dosage/Route** | • For scabies, apply thin layer of cream or lotion over entire skin surface from the neck down. After 8 to 12 hours, wash drug off. Repeat in 1 week if mites appear or new lesions develop. |

Permethrin

Description	• Scabicide
Indications	• Scabies
Contraindications	• Allergy to pyrethrins, pyrethroids, or chrysanthemums
Precautions	• Avoid eyes; pregnancy category B
	• Adverse reactions: Pruritus, burning, stinging, tingling, numbness, erythema, rash
Dosage/Route	• Massage into skin from head to soles of feet. Remove 8 to 14 hours later by washing. Usually one treatment suffices; if living mites are present after 14 days, re-treat.

Povidone Iodine (Betadine)

Description	• Mild skin cleanser
Indications	• Provides residual protection against future bacterial infection
Contraindications	• Known allergy to iodine
Precautions	• Adverse reactions: Local irritation
Dosage/Route	• Apply to IV or preoperative site; allow to air dry.

Sebutone/Sebulex Shampoo

Description	• Antiseborrheic
Indications	• Adjuncts in the treatment of dandruff and seborrheic dermatitis to relieve itching and scaling of the scalp
Contraindications	• Known hypersensitivity to ingredients
Precautions	• None
Dosage/Route	• Apply to wet scalp and lather, let stay for 10 minutes, then rinse thoroughly; repeat two to three times per week.

Topical Anesthetics (Nupercainal/Dibucaine Ointment)

Description	• Topical pain reliever
Indications	• Provides temporary relief of pain and itching from hemorrhoid by lubricating dry and inflamed skin. May also be used for sunburn, minor cuts, and burns.
Contraindications	• None
Precautions	• Do not use in or near the eyes.
Dosage/Route	• Apply to affected area as needed.

Visine Eye Drops

| **Description** | • Ophthalmic vasoconstrictor |
| **Indications** | • Provides relief for tired and irritated eyes resulting from dilated blood vessels |

Contraindications	• Known hypersensitivity or glaucoma
Precautions	• Rebound may occur with frequent or prolonged use.
Dosage/Route	• Instill 1 to 2 drops up to four times daily.

Zinc Oxide Ointment

Description	• Anti-irritant
Indications	• Provides temporary relief of minor skin irritations and provides a protective coating for inflamed tissues
Contraindications	• None
Precautions	• None
Dosage/Route	• Apply to affected area as needed.

Upper Respiratory Infection Medications

Afrin Nasal Spray

Description	• Nasal decongestant
Indications	• Nasal congestion
Contraindications	• Patients hypersensitive to the drug
Precautions	• Adverse reactions ▪ Central nervous system: Headache, anxiety, restlessness, dizziness, insomnia ▪ Cardiovascular: Palpitations, cardiovascular collapse, hypertension ▪ EENT: Rebound nasal congestion or irritation, dryness of nose and throat, increased nasal discharge, stinging, sneezing • Considerations ▪ Use cautiously in patients with hyperthyroidism, cardiac disease, hypertension, or diabetes.
Dosage/Route	• Two to three sprays in each nostril twice daily. Use no longer than 3 to 5 days.

Cepacol Lozenges

Description	• Throat lozenge
Indications	• Throat irritation
Contraindications	• None
Precautions	• None
Dosage/Route	• Let one troche dissolve in mouth as needed.

Chloraseptic Gargle

Description	• Topical throat analgesic
Indications	• Provides soothing relief from throat irritations
Contraindications	• None
Precautions	• None
Dosage/Route	• Spray or gargle every 3 to 4 hours as needed.

Dextromethorphan

Description	• Nonnarcotic antitussive activity comparable to that of codeine but less likely to cause codeine symptoms

	(i.e., constipation, drowsiness, or gastrointestinal disturbances)
Indications	• Temporary relief of cough spasms in nonproductive coughs due to colds, pertussis, and influenza
Contraindications	• Asthma, productive cough, persistent or chronic cough, hepatic function impairment
Precautions	• Chronic pulmonary disease, patients on MAO inhibitors, and patients with an enlarged prostrate
Dosage/Route	• Adult, oral: 10-20 mg every 4 hours, or 30 mg every 6 to 8 hours (maximum 120 mg daily); or 60 mg of the sustained-action liquid twice daily.

Entex

Description	• Decongestant plus expectorant
Indications	• Congestion
Contraindications	• Severe hypertension, coronary artery disease
Precautions	• Hypertension, diabetes, cardiovascular disease, glaucoma, gastrointestinal or urinary obstruction
Dosage/Route	• One capsule every 12 hours

Pseudoephedrine Hydrochloride (Sudafed)

Description	• Decongestant
Indications	• Symptomatic relief of nasal congestion associated with rhinitis and sinusitis; eustachian tube congestion
Contraindications	• Hypersensitivity to Sudafed • Severe hypertension • Coronary artery disease • Glaucoma • Hyperthyroidism or patients taking MAO inhibitors

Precautions	• Side effects
	  ▪ Transient restlessness
	  ▪ Stimulation
	  ▪ Tachycardia
	  ▪ Nervousness
	  ▪ Dizziness
	  ▪ Dry mouth
	• Considerations
	  ▪ Drug may act as a stimulant.
	  ▪ Avoid taking within 2 hours of bedtime.
	  ▪ Advise patient to stop taking medication if extreme restlessness occurs and to consult MD or PA.
	  ▪ Advise patients that many over-the-counter drugs may contain ephedrine or other sympathomimetic amines and might intensify the action of pseudoephedrine if taken together.

Dosage/Route	• Adults: 30-60 mg orally every 4 to 6 hours; maximum daily dose (24-hour period) is 240 mg.

Tessalon Perles

Description	• Antitussive
Indications	• Symptomatic relief of cough
Contraindications	• Hypersensitivity to drug or related compounds
Precautions	• Adverse reactions: Headache, sedation, tachycardia, dizziness, gastrointestinal upset, dizziness, pruritus, skin eruptions
Dosage/Route	• 100-200 mg three times daily. Swallow whole—do not suck or chew.

Volume Expansion

Hetastarch (Hextend)

Description	• Plasma volume expander, fluid replacement
Indications	• Severe bleeding; fluid replacement
Contraindications	• Patients with known hypersensitivity to drug; renal failure with oliguria or anuria; severe heart failure
Precautions	• Adverse reactions: Metabolic—fluid overload. • Considerations: Use cautiously in patients with heart failure, circulatory insufficiency, renal dysfunction, or pulmonary edema.
Dosage/Route	• 500 mL of 6% hetastarch (Hextend; weighs 1.3 lb) will expand the intravascular volume by 800 mL within 1 hour. After hemorrhage is controlled to the extent possible, start 500 mL of Hextend. If mental status improves and radial pulse returns, maintain saline lock and hold fluids. If no response is seen within 30 minutes, give an additional 500 mL of Hextend and monitor vital signs.

Lactated Ringer's

Description	• Fluid and electrolyte replacement
Indications	• Fluid and electrolyte replacement
Contraindications	• Patients with renal failure, except as emergency volume expander
Precautions	• Adverse reactions: Metabolic—electrolyte imbalance, fluid overload. • Considerations: Use cautiously in patients with heart failure, circulatory insufficiency, renal dysfunction, or pulmonary edema.
Dosage/Route	• Highly individualized. May need bolus of 1 to 2 liters depending on indication; usually 1.5 to 3 liters infused IV over 18 to 24 hours maintenance.

Miscellaneous

Fostex Soap

Description	• Cleanser
Indications	• Used in the treatment of acne, dandruff, and other skin conditions characterized by excessive oil production

Contraindications	· None
Precautions	· None
Dosage/Route	· Use as needed.

Hydrogen Peroxide

Description	· Cleanser for the skin
Indications	· To control bacterial infection. It may also be used as a gargle (full strength or diluted with water) for relief of throat discomfort.
Contraindications	· None
Precautions	· None
Dosage/Route	· Use as needed.

Lidocaine Hydrochloride (Xylocaine)

Description	· Local anesthetic administered parenterally by injection
Indications	· To provide local anesthesia for wound care, laceration repair, and/or other minor superficial surgical procedures; peripheral nerve block
Contraindications	· Hypersensitivity, severe liver disease
Precautions	· Adverse reactions (side effects) ▪ Central nervous system: Anxiety, disorientation, seizures, shivering, tremors, loss of consciousness ▪ Cardiovascular: Bradycardia, cardiac arrest, dysrhythmias, myocardial depression, hypotension, hypertension ▪ Gastrointestinal: Nausea, vomiting ▪ EENT: Blurred vision, tinnitus, pupil constriction ▪ Respiratory: Respiratory arrest, status asthmaticus, anaphylaxis ▪ Skin: Allergic reactions, burning, edema, irritation, rash, tissue necrosis, urticaria · Available with and without epinephrine; *do not use epinephrine on digits, ears, nose, or penis.*

Prednisone

Description	· Glucocorticoid
Indications	· Severe inflammation, steroid-responsive disorders
Contraindications	· Systemic fungal infections, known hypersensitivity to the drug
Precautions	· Masks infection. · Adverse reactions: Euphoria, insomnia, psychotic behavior, heart failure, hypertension, edema, arrhythmias, gastrointestinal irritation, peptic ulceration, pancreatitis. After abrupt withdrawal: Rebound inflammation, fatigue, weakness, arthralgia, fever, dizziness, lethargy, depression, fainting.
Dosage/Route	· Dosage is individualized. 5-60 mg orally daily in a single dose or as two to four divided doses.

Training
91W Life Cycle

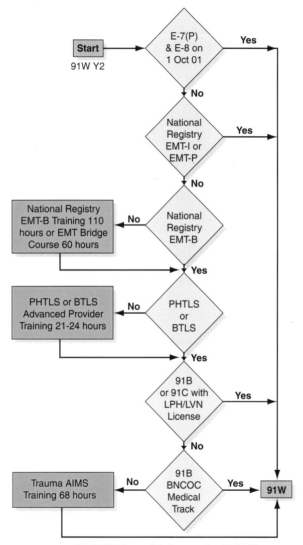

RC BNCOC completed on or after 10-01-01

Figure 35 91W life cycle.

Rank	AMEDD Course Number	Training	Length	Location	Attendance Requirement	Self-Development Course Number	Self-Development	Length	Location	Attendance Requirement
E1-E5	750-BT	Basic Combat Training	9 weeks	Ft. LW/Ft. Still/Ft. Jackson/Ft. Benning	IET		Professional Postgraduate Short Course Program			
	300-91W10	Health Care Specialist	16 weeks	FSH, TX	AIT/MOS	300-A0704	75/71 Personnel/Retention Legal/EO	4 days	SA, TX	Sustainment
		See ASIs N#, N(PI, P2, P3, M6, M3, Y6				340-A0715	MEDCOM CSV/SGM SR NCO	4 days	SA, TX	Sustainment
	600-PLDC	Primary Leadership Development Course (PLDC)	4 weeks	Multiple sites	Leadership	340-A0743	CSM/SGM SR NCO Course	4 days	Landstuhl, Germany	Sustainment
	5H-F5/302-F5	Flight Medic Course	4 weeks	Ft. Rucker, AL	Voluntary SQI F	6A-300/A0130	Joint Services Emergency Medicine Symposium	5 days	SA, TX	Sustainment
		Ranger Medical NCO Course	52 weeks	Ft. Benning, GA	Voluntary ASI WI	6E-300/A0502	Annual Field Medicine Short Course	3 days	Ft. Sam Houston, TX	Sustainment
	600-BNCOC	NCO Basic (Common Core) Ph1	2 weeks, 2 days	Multiple sites	DA Selection Leadership	6H-300/A0406	Sperandio, Plans Operations, Intelligence, Training	5 days	Ft. Sam Houston, TX	Sustainment
	400-BNCOC(F)	NCO Basic (Common Core) Ph1 (TATS)	2 weeks, 2 days	Multiple sites	DA Selection Leadership		Correspondence Course			
	6-8-C40 (91W30)	AMEDD NCO Basic (NCOES) Ph2 (Transition completed)	7 weeks, 4 days	Ft. Sam Houston, TX	DA Selection Leadership	081-CBRNE-W	Introduction to CBRNE		Online	JIT-Prereq for PPSCPs
	6-8-C40 (91WY2)	AMEDD NCO Basic (NCOES) Ph2 (Transition required)	14 weeks, 4 days	Ft. Sam Houston, TX	DA Selection Leadership					
E6-E7	5K-F3/520-F3	Instructor Training Course	2 weeks	AHS	JIT/SI (5K)		Specialty Courses			
	5K-F6/520-F6	Small Group Instructor Training Course (SGITC)	1 week	AHS	JIT	5K-F13/520-F10	CBRNE Trainer Evaluation	2 days	Ft. Sam Houston, TX	JIT/CHE
	250-ASI2S	Battle Staff NCO	4 weeks, 1 day	USASMA (Ft. Bliss)	JIT ASI 2S	5K-F5/520-F5-(OATP)	Orientation to the AMEDD Training Process	2 days	Ft. Sam Houston, TX	JIT

Rank	AMEDD Course Number	Training	Length	Location	Attendance Requirement	Self-Development Course Number	Self-Development	Length	Location	Attendance Requirement
	501-SQI4	Recruiter	7 weeks, 4 days	USAREC	JIT SQI 4	5K-F7/520-F7	Advanced Instructor Training Course (Ph 1 and 2)	1 week, 3 days	Ft. Sam Houston, TX	JIT
	012-SQIX	Drill Sgt. School	9 weeks	Multiple sites	JIT SQI-X		Air Assault School	2 weeks	Ft. Campbell, various sites	Once/upon assignment to Air Assault position/voluntary
		Inspector General NCO				2E-SI5P/SQI7/001-SQIP	Airborne Training	3 weeks	Ft. Benning	Once/upon assignment to Air Assault position/voluntary
		Equal Opportunity Advisor					EMT-Intermediate		Various locations	
		Reserve Component Advisor					EMT-Paramedic		Various locations	
		Observer/Controller CT								
	600-ANCOC	NCO Advanced (Common Core) Ph1	2 weeks, 2 days	Multiple sites	DA Selection Leadership					
	400-ANCOC (F)	NCO Advanced (Common Core) PH1 (TATS)	2 weeks, 2 days	Multiple sites	DA Selection Leadership					
	6-8-C42	AMEDD NCO Advanced (NCOES) Ph2	2 weeks, 2 days	Ft. Sam Houston, TX	DA Selection Leadership					
	TC-8-800	Semi-Annual Combat Medical Skills Validation Test		Unit Training	Semi-Annual					
		Emergency Medical Technician-Basic		Multiple sites	Re-certification (every two years)					
E8	521-SQIM	First Sergeant Course Ph1/Ph2	Ph1-DL, Ph2-3 weeks	USASMA	JIT SQI-M					
E9	1-250-C5	U.S. Army Sergeants Major Course	38 weeks, 2 days	USASMA (Ft. Bliss)	DA Selection					
	521-F1	Command Sergeant Major Course	1 week	USASMA	Leadership					

NOTE: Convert a to 9IZ at SGM

Continuing Education Tracking Sheet

Title of Class/ Course	Date	Instructor/Unit	Continuing Education Hours

Scope of Practice

Job Description

To provide patient assessment, teaching, emergency care, and nursing care within the medical treatment facility (MTF). As a foundation, the Health Care Specialist will maintain the skills of a National Registry–certified emergency medical technician–basic (EMT-B), to include basic life support (BLS).

Military Course

Phase 1: AMEDDC&S, Fort Sam Houston, TX; the Army School System (TASS) BN, USARC Regions A–G
- Course length
  - Initial entry training, active component (AC): 16 weeks
  - Reclassification training, Reserve component (RC): To be determined
- Accreditation: National accreditation from the National Registry of Emergency Medical Technicians (NREMT)
- American Council on Education credit hours: Pending
- School affiliation: None
- Degree awarded: None
- Eligibility for certification or licensing: Trainees are required to take and pass the EMT-B certification examination administered by NREMT.

Clinical Baseline Competency Task List

- Procedures requiring direct supervision
  - Assists licensed and/or privileged providers to perform invasive procedures. Sets up and maintains a sterile field.
  - Assists in emergency childbirth.
  - Per nursing protocol or per physician order, administers, records, and evaluates response to the following medications: nitroglycerin sublingually, activated charcoal, oral and/or IV glucose, and beta-agonist metered dose inhaler or nebulizer.
  - Performs proper airway management for respiratory distress, including placement of a Combitube. Note: Does not include endo-tracheal intubation.
  - Inserts and monitors nasogastric tube for content, output, and position and performs gastric lavage as instructed.
- Procedures requiring indirect supervision
  - Patient assessment
    - Performs and documents general physical assessment and level of consciousness.
    - Performs triage per protocol.

- Obtains, interprets, and documents temperature, heart rate, respiratory rate, pulse oximetry, and blood pressure and reports deviations from normal.
- Obtains and documents basic patient history, including medication history, prior surgery, social history, allergies, and past medical problems.
- Assesses visual acuity with eye chart and assesses gross hearing function.
- Performs 12-lead electrocardiogram; places patient on cardiac monitor.
- Obtains laboratory specimens, including blood (venipuncture, capillary), urine, and cultures (wound, stool, urine, throat, sputum, and blood).
- Monitors and records intake and output and the appearance of output.
- Interventions
  - Initiates, monitors, and discontinues intravenous infusion or saline lock.
  - Controls bleeding by applying pressure bandages, pressure points, and splints.
  - Utilizes proper technique in the initial management of fractures and initiates spinal precautions in suspected spinal injuries.
  - Assists in the initial treatment of an environmental injury.
  - Performs, interprets, records, and reports fingerstick blood glucose monitoring.
  - Recognizes indications for, provides, and monitors by clinical assessment and pulse oximetry the use of supplemental oxygen via nasal cannula, oxygen mask, pocket mask, or bag-valve-mask device.
  - Performs ear and eye irrigation.
  - Per provider order, administers and records appropriate immunizations. Note: Does not include skin testing or allergy desensitization shots.
  - Performs appropriate wound care using sterile technique, including dressing changes, wound cultures, and wound irrigation.
  - Per nursing protocol, administers and records oral and rectal medications in a clinical setting.

Related Civilian Equivalent Training

- Course length: EMT-B, 110 hours minimum
- Degree awarded: None

- Areas of clinical competency: Reference the cognitive, affective, and psychomotor skills identified by the U.S. Department of Transportation EMT-Basic National Standard Curriculum

Licensing and Credentialing

- Army standard or requirement(s) for licensure and/or certification: NREMT-B certification and health care provider cardiopulmonary resuscitation (CPR)
- National and state requirement: None
- Degree requirements: None
- Licensing and/or certification examination: NREMT-B

Continuing Education Requirements

- Army standard or requirements(s) for licensure and/or certification: Must retain NREMT-B recertification requirements.
- Maintain civilian license and/or certification: The following list identifies the EMT-B recertification requirements.
  - Continuing education hours: 40 hours every 2 years; requirements outlined by NREMT. Must submit continuing education hours with recertification packet to National Registry.
  - Refresher course: 24 hours every 2 years; complete toward the end of the second year.
  - Skills verification: 4 hours every 2 years; complete in conjunction with refresher course.
  - Health provider CPR: 8 hours every 2 years. Required certification to maintain NREMT.

Military Occupational Specialty Requirement and NREMT Certification

- Soldiers (AC/RC) possessing the 91W military occupational specialty (MOS) are required to obtain and maintain certification by the NREMT. Certification will be at the basic level (EMT-B), and those who are EMT-B, I (Intermediate), or P (Paramedic) must maintain recertification every 2 years. For MEDCOM, the Semi-Annual Combat Medic Skills Validation Test (SACMSVT) must be completed every 6 months.
- Soldiers who fail to recertify according to NREMT guidance will be granted an additional 90 calendar days (for AC) or 180 calendar days (for RC) to obtain NREMT-B certification; soldiers will be deemed MOS qualified during this period. A soldier's failure to obtain NREMT certification immediately following the respective 90- or 180-day period will result in a status of non-MOS-qualified (MOSQ) and the initiation of appropriate personnel action (i.e., mandatory reclassification, separation according to governing regulations).

STP 8-9W15-SM-TG

Field Expedient Squad Book Mos 91 W

Name	Semi-Annually/Annually STP 8-9W15-SM-TG 10 October 2001	Date					
Task Number and Short Title **Skill Level 1-5 Vital Signs**		**Status**					
		T-P-U	T-P-U	T-P-U	T-P-U	T-P-U	T-P-U
081-831-0010	Measure a patient's respirations/Semi-annually						
081-831-0011	Measure a patient's pulse/ Semi-annually						
081-831-0012	Measure a patient's blood pressure/Semi-annually						
081-831-0013	Measure a patient's temperature/Semi-annually						
081-833-0164	Measure a patient's pulse oxygen saturation/ Semi-annually						
Emergency Medical Treatment							
081-831-0018	Open the airway/ Semi-annually						
081-831-0019	Clear an upper airway obstruction/Semi-annually						
081-831-0046	Administer external chest compressions/Semi-annually						
081-831-0048	Perform rescue breathing/ Semi-annually						
081-833-0161	Control bleeding/ Semi-annually						
081-833-0167	Place a patient on a cardiac monitor/Semi-annually						
081-833-3027	Manage cardiac arrest using AED/Semi-annually						
Skill Level 1-5 Basic Medical Care							
081-831-0007	Perform a patient care handwash/Semi-annually						
081-831-0008	Put on sterile gloves/ Semi-annually						
081-831-0033	Initiate a field medical card/ Annually						
081-833-0076	Apply restraining devices to patients/Annually						
081-833-0006	Measure a patient's intake and output/Annually						
081-833-0007	Establish a sterile field/ Annually						
081-833-0010	Change a sterile dressing/ Annually						
081-833-0012	Perform a wound irrigation/ Annually						

Task Number and Short Title	Status					
Skill Level 1-5 Basic Medical Care	T-P-U	T-P-U	T-P-U	T-P-U	T-P-U	T-P-U
081-833-0021 Perform oral and nasopharyngeal suctioning of a patient/Semi-annually						
081-833-0059 Irrigate an obstructed ear/ Annually						
081-833-0145 Document patient care using subjective, objective, assessment, plan (SOAP) note format/Annually						
081-833-0165 Perform patient hygiene/ Annually						
081-835-3007 Obtain an electrocardiogram/Annually						
Skill Level 1-5 Respiratory Dysfunction/Airway Management						
081-833-0016 Insert an oropharyngeal airway (J Tube)/ Semi-annually						
081-833-0018 Set up an oxygen tank/ Semi-annually						
081-833-0142 Insert a nasopharyngeal airway/Semi-annually						
081-833-0158 Administer oxygen/ Semi-annually						
081-833-0169 Insert a Combitube/ Semi-annually						
081-833-3006 Perform a needle cricothyroidotomy/Annually						
081-833-3007 Perform needle chest decompression/ Semi-annually						
Venipuncture and IV Therapy						
081-833-0032 Obtain a blood specimen using a vacutainer/Annually						
081-833-0033 Initiate an intravenous infusion/Semi-annually						
081-833-0034 Manage a patient with an intravenous infusion/ Semi-annually						
081-835-3025 Initiate a saline lock/ Annually						
Skill Level 1-5 Casualty Management						
081-831-0035 Manage a convulsive and/or seizing patient/Annually						
081-833-0045 Treat a casualty with an open abdominal wound/ Annually						
081-833-0046 Apply a dressing to an impalement injury/Annually						
081-833-0048 Manage an unconscious casualty/Annually						
081-833-0049 Treat a casualty with a closed chest wound/Annually						

Task Number and Short Title Skill Level 1-5 Casualty Management		Status					
		T-P-U	T-P-U	T-P-U	T-P-U	T-P-U	T-P-U
081-833-0050	Treat a casualty with an open chest wound/Annually						
081-833-0052	Treat a casualty with an open or closed head injury/ Annually						
081-833-0070	Administer initial treatment for burns/Annually						
081-833-0103	Provide care for a soldier with symptoms of battle fatigue/Annually						
081-833-0116	Assist in vaginal delivery/ Annually						
081-833-0143	Treat a poisoned casualty/ Annually						
081-833-0144	Treat a diabetic emergency/ Annually						
081-833-0155	Perform a trauma casualty assessment/Semi-annually						
081-833-0156	Perform a medical patient assessment/Semi-annually						
081-833-0159	Treat a cardiac emergency/ Annually						
081-833-0160	Treat a respiratory emergency/Annually						
081-835-3030	Determine a patient's level of consciousness using the Glasgow coma scale/Annually						
	Eye Injuries						
081-833-0054	Irrigate eyes/Annually						
081-833-0056	Treat foreign bodies of the eye/Annually						
081-833-0057	Treat lacerations, contusions, and extrusions of the eye/Annually						
081-833-0058	Treat burns of the eye/ Annually						
	Skill Level 1-4 Skeletal Dysfunction						
081-831-0044	Apply a pneumatic splint to a casualty with a suspected fracture of an extremity/ Annually						
081-833-0060	Apply a roller bandage/ Annually						
081-833-0062	Immobilize a suspected fracture of the arm or dislocated shoulder/Annually						
081-833-0064	Immbolize a suspected dislocated or fractured hip/ Annually						
081-833-0092	Transport a casualty with a suspected spinal injury/ Semi-annually						

Task Number and Short Title	Status					
Skill Level 1-4 Skeletal Dysfunction	T-P-U	T-P-U	T-P-U	T-P-U	T-P-U	T-P-U
081-833-0141	Apply a traction splint/ Semi-annually						
081-833-0154	Provide basic emergency treatment for a painful, swollen, deformed extremity/ Annually						
Environmental Injuries							
081-831-0038	Treat a casualty for a heat injury/Annually						
081-831-0039	Treat a casualty for a cold injury/Annually						
081-833-0031	Initiate treatment for anaphylactic shock/Annually						
081-833-0072	Treat a casualty for insect bites or stings/Annually						
081-833-0073	Treat a casualty for snakebite/Annually						
Shock							
081-833-0047	Initiate treatment for hypovolemic shock/ Semi-annually						
081-833-3011	Apply pneumatic anti-shock garment/Annually						
Skill Level 1-5 Chemical Agent Injuries							
081-833-0083	Treat a nerve agent casualty in the field/Semi-annually						
081-833-0084	Treat a blood agent (hydrogen cyanide) casualty in the field/Semi-annually						
081-833-0085	Treat a choking agent casualty in the field/ Semi-annually						
081-833-0086	Treat a blister agent casualty (mustard, Lewisite, phosgene oxime) in the field/ Semi-annually						
081-833-0095	Decontaminate a casualty/ Annually						
Urinary Catheterization							
081-833-3017	Insert a urinary catheter/ Annually						
081-835-3010	Maintain an indwelling urinary catheter/Annually						
Gastric Intubation							
081-833-3022	Insert a nasogastric tube/ Annually						
081-835-3005	Perform a gastric lavage/ Annually						
Force Protection/Risk Assessment							
081-831-0037	Disinfect water for drinking/ Annually						

Task Number and Short Title Skill Level 1-4 Triage and Evacuation	Status					
	T-P-U	T-P-U	T-P-U	T-P-U	T-P-U	T-P-U
071-334-4001 Guide a helicopter to a landing point/Annually						
071-334-4002 Establish a helicopter landing point/Annually						
081-833-0080 Triage casualties on a conventional battlefield/ Semi-annually						
081-833-0082 Triage casualties on an integrated battlefield/ Semi-annually						
081-833-0151 Load casualties onto ground evacuation platforms/ Annually						
081-833-0171 Load casualties onto nonstandard vehicles, 1¼ ton, 4x4, M998/Annually						
081-833-0172 Load casualties onto nonstandard vehicles, 2½ ton, 6x6 or 5 ton, 6x6, cargo truck /Annually						
081-833-0173 Load casualties onto nonstandard vehicles, 5 ton M-1085, M-1093, 2½ ton M-1081/Annually						
Skill Level 1-5 Medication Administration						
081-833-0088 Prepare an injection for administration/Annually						
081-833-0089 Administer an injection (intramuscular, subcutaneous, intradermal)/Annually						
081-833-0174 Administer morphine/ Semi-annually						
081-835-3001 Administer oral medications/ Annually						
081-835-3020 Administer topical medications/Annually						
081-835-3021 Administer rectal or vaginal medications/Annually						
081-835-3022 Administer medicated eye drops or ointments/Annually						
Skill Level 2-5 Advanced Procedures (SL 2)						
081-833-0170 Perform endotracheal suctioning of a patient/ Annually						
081-835-3024 Provide tracheostomy care/Annually						
081-835-3031 Provide nursing care for a patient with a waterseal drainage system/Annually						

Task Number and Short Title Skill Level 3-5 Advanced Procedures (SL 3)		Status					
		T-P-U	T-P-U	T-P-U	T-P-U	T-P-U	T-P-U
081-830-3016	Intubate a patient/Annually						
081-833-0093	Set up a casualty decontamination station/ Annually						
081-833-0168	Insert a chest tube/Annually						
081-833-3005	Perform a surgical cricothyroidotomy/Annually						
081-833-3014	Perform a neurological examination on a patient with suspected central nervous system (CNS) injuries/Annually						
081-835-3000	Administer blood/Annually						
081-835-3002	Administer medications by IV piggyback/Annually						
081-833-3208	Suture a minor laceration/ Annually						

STP 8-9W15 −SM-TG Soldier's Manual, Skill Levels 1/2/3/4/5 and Trainer's Guide, MOS 91W, Health Care Specialist 10 October 2001

Combat Lifesaver Program Correspondence Course Option

○ Points of contact: If you have any questions about enrollment or graduation status, please contact the Army Institute for Professional Development by calling DSN 826-2127/3322 or Commercial (757) 878-2127/3322. Send e-mail to sectiona@atsc.army.mil. You can also write to the following address:

> The Army Institute for Professional Development
> Attn. ATIC-ATIC-DLS (Section A)
> U.S. Army Training Support Center
> Fort Eustis, Virginia 23628-0001

If you have any questions about the content of the Combat Lifesaver Program, please contact Mr. Don Atkerson:

> Academy of Health Sciences
> Multimedia Development Branch
> Attn. MCCS HLD
> 2250 Stanley Road (Room 315)
> Fort Sam Houston, Texas 78234-6130
> DSN: 471-7330 or Commercial: (210) 221-7330
> E-mail: don.atkerson@cen.amedd.army.milL

The Combat Lifesaver

The Army battle doctrine was developed for a widely dispersed, rapidly moving battlefield. Battlefield constraints will limit the ability of trained medical personnel to provide immediate, far forward care. Therefore, the combat lifesaver (CL) program was developed to provide the needed additional care to combat casualties.

The CL is a bridge between the self-aid/buddy-aid (SABA) training given to all soldiers during basic training and the medical training given to the combat medic/health care specialist. The CL is a nonmedical soldier trained to provide emergency care as a secondary mission. He or she does not replace the combat medic. The primary mission of the CL is the combat mission. Each squad, crew, team, or equivalent-sized element should have at least one member trained as a CL. Medical units that have organic clinical and/or treatment personnel assigned are exempt from this requirement, but may choose to train some personnel to support the mission. The CL will provide care to members of his or her squad, team, or crew as the mission permits. When the CL has no combat mission to perform, the CL may assist the combat medic in providing far forward care and in preparing casualties for evacuation. Information concerning the role of the CL can be found in Chapter 12 of Army Regulation 350-41, Training in Units.

Introduction to the Combat Lifesaver Course

The Combat Lifesaver Course (CLC) is designed to be used by both active duty and Reserve component students. The "D" edition is the most current edition. Previous editions are obsolete.

The CLC is offered through correspondence, utilizing the group study mode. Classroom instruction takes place under qualified medical instructors such as senior medical NCOs selected by the unit commander. Students who successfully complete all written and performance examinations will receive 40 credit hours (8 promotion points for enlisted personnel) and be recognized as CLs.

- Duration: The CLC can be conducted in 3 days of group training time. Students study subcourses IS0824 and IS0825 before coming to class. Day 1 consists of testing all SABA tasks (IS0824). Days 2 and 3 concentrate on teaching and testing the medical tasks (IS0825) that are beyond the level of SABA care.
- Contents: The CLC consists of two student subcourse texts (Interschool Subcourses 0824 and 0825), a student examination booklet, and an instructor's manual (Interschool Subcourse 0826). Subcourse 0826 also contains the performance examination used to

fulfill the requirement that combat lifesavers be retested (recertified) every 12 months.

Administrative Instructions

The following guidelines are given to help you administer the CLC.

○ Arrange for equipment and supplies: Make arrangements to obtain all of the equipment and supplies that you will need to conduct the course as early as possible. Certain items (such as IV trainers and rescue breathing manikins) may need to be purchased. Check with your local Training Visual Information Support Center (T/VISC) concerning these items. A suggested list of equipment and supplies needed for 10 students is given later in this section. Modify the list as needed to make sure that enough equipment and supplies will be available for the course. None of this equipment will be provided by the Army Institute for Professional Development (AIPD) or by the U.S. Army Medical Department Center and School. You must obtain them through your own procurement system.

○ Enroll students and instructor(s): The request for enrollment sent to AIPD must contain (1) a cover letter, (2) a DA Form 145 enrolling the primary instructor (group leader) in ISO826, and (3) a student roster. The cover letter should be signed by the battalion commander or by a lieutenant colonel or higher. The roster must include each student's name, rank, Social Security number, component code, and RYE date, if applicable. All subcourse materials (students' subcourses, examination booklets, response sheets, and instructor's manual) will be sent to the primary instructor. The roster must also include the name and Social Security number of the primary instructor. It is recommended that you send the enrollment applications to AIPD at least 6 weeks before group instruction is to begin. Overseas locations should allow additional time. Additional enrollment information can be found in DA Pamphlet 350-59, Army Correspondence Course Program Catalog.

○ Obtain instructor(s) and assistant instructor(s): Estimate the number and types of instructor(s) and assistant(s) that will be needed. The primary instructor must be at least a senior medical NCO (see paragraph 12, AR 350-41; and DA Pamphlet 350-59, page 16, Section VIII, paragraph 2-51). The instructor for the intravenous infusion lesson must be an expert in administering IVs and also be qualified to handle emergencies that could arise when students practice initiating IVs on each other. Additional suggestions concerning the instructor(s) and assistant(s) can be found in ISO826.

- Reserve facilities: Reserve the facilities needed for the course. The facilities should allow the students to clearly see the demonstrations and provide plenty of room for student practice. Make sure that enough tables and chairs will be available.
- Check AIPD materials: When you receive the materials from AIPD, read the introductory material in the instructor's manual (IS0826). This subcourse lists the materials that you should have received. It also provides you with lesson plans for all of the tasks covered in the CLC. Instructions are provided for administering performance and written examination, retesting students, and testing students annually for recertification. Procedures for dropping students and for substituting students are also given in the subcourse.
- Give subcourses to students: If possible, give each student a set of student subcourses (IS0824 and IS0825) about 2 weeks before the classroom instruction begins. *Do not give out the examination booklets.* This should give the student sufficient time to read and study the subcourses. If the students are already familiar with the lesson material when they come to class, the instructor can devote more time to demonstrations, discussions, and student practice. If possible, provide each student with a field first aid dressing and two muslin bandages when you distribute the subcourses. This will allow the students to practice some of the tasks before being tested on the SABA tasks.
  - Interschool Subcourse 0824 Edition D, Combat Lifesaver Course: Buddy-Aid Tasks
  - Interschool Subcourse 0825 Edition D, Combat Lifesaver Course: Medical Tasks
  - Interschool Subcourse 0826 Edition D, Combat Lifesaver Course: Instructor's Manual; contains lesson plans for all of the tasks, a copy of each performance checklist, solution sheets to the written examinations, and a copy of the recertification examination

> **note**
>
> Solutions to written examinations are not included in the downloads.

The Student Examination Booklet contains one copy of each performance checklist, four written (multiple-choice) examinations (versions 1 and 2 for subcourse IS0824 and versions 1 and 2 for subcourse IS0825), and a recertification examination for later use.

Quantity	Nomenclature	Federal Stock Number	Unit of Issue
1	Case med inst and supply set	6545-00-912-9870	EA
14	Tube drain 1 3 18, (can be used for tourniquet), 200s	6515-01-188-5316	PG
1	Intravenous injection set (48)	6515-00-115-0032	PG
50/200	Catheter and needle unit, IV 18 gauge, disposable	6515-01-315-6227	PG
3	Ringer's injection lactated, 500 mL (18)	6505-01-462-3022	PG
1	Gloves (50 pairs)	6515-00-226-7692	PG
10	Scissors, bandage, angular, 7.25 inch	6515-00-935-7138	EA
10	Adhesive tape, 1" × 10 yds	6510-00-926-8882	SL
60	Dressing, first aid, field, camouflaged, 4 × 7	6510-00-159-4883	EA
120	Bandage, muslin, OD, 37 × 37 × 52	6510-00-201-1755	EA
1	Pad, povidone-iodine impregnated (100)	6510-01-010-0307	BX
5	Poncho, nylon	8405-01-100-0096	EA
4	Litter, folding	6530-00-783-7205	EA
1	Manikin, resuscitation (Resusci-Anne), or other rescue breathing trainer	6910-01-206-0312	EA
5	Training device, IV, arm (or similar device)	6910-01-080-2884	EA
1	Pad, isopropyl alcohol	6510-00-786-3736	PG
6	Hypodermic, autoinjector, demonstration	6910-01-061-6444	BX
1	Sponge, surgical, 2 × 2	6510-01-464-0826	PG
1	Splint, universal, malleable, 36" × 4.5", 12s	6515-01-255-4681	PG
1	Canteen, 1 quart, plastic	8464-01-115-0026	EA
1	Protective mask with hood		EA
1	Pair of chemical protective gloves		PR
1	Basin (used during decontamination of blister agent)		EA
1	Vehicle (used to demonstrate loading casualties)		EA
	Rope (used to secure litters to vehicle, if needed)		FT
#	Blanket, wool	7200-00-715-7985	EA
#	Holder, nerve agent training device antidote kit (Mark I)	6530-01-141-7458	PG

continued

#	CANA kit training device	6910-01-275-4833	PG
#	Skin decontaminating kit, M291	4230-01-276-1905	BX
#	Water purification tablets, iodine	6850-00-986-7166	BT
#	DEET, 71% diethyltoluamide, 2 oz (insect repellent in plastic bottle)	6840-00-753-4963	BT
#	DEET, 71% diethyltoluamide, 6 oz (insect repellent in aerosol can)	6840-00-082-2541	CN
#	Grease pencils		EA
#	Stick-like objects (for tourniquets)		EA
#	Poles (for improvised litters)		EA
#	Jackets or shirts (for improvised litter)		EA
#	Boards or other rigid objects for forearm/leg splints		EA
#	Old boots (1 pair for stabilizing suspected neck injury)		PR
#	Wooden pole (for removing electrical wire)		EA
#	Poncho, backpack, or other devices for elevating legs		EA
#	Old shirts and trousers (worn by simulated casualty and cut during demonstration)		EA
#	Material for padding splints, improvised cravats, and bandages		N/A

Training Scenarios

Scenario 1

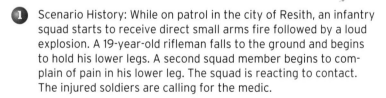

1 Scenario History: While on patrol in the city of Resith, an infantry squad starts to receive direct small arms fire followed by a loud explosion. A 19-year-old rifleman falls to the ground and begins to hold his lower legs. A second squad member begins to complain of pain in his lower leg. The squad is reacting to contact. The injured soldiers are calling for the medic.

2 Injuries

○ Patient 1
  ■ Partial amputation to the left lower leg at boot-top level
  ■ Multiple fragmentary wounds to right lower leg

- Patient 2
  - Fragmentary wound to right lower leg

3 Moulage Instructions

- Patient 1
  - Manikin has left lower leg partial amputation with arterial bleeding (leg removed at hinge).
  - Right lower leg has five 1- to 2-mm puncture wounds with small amount of bleeding.
- Patient 2
  - Small tear in BDU pants
  - Two 1- to 2-mm puncture wounds to right lower leg with minimal bleeding

4 Patient 2 Instructions

- You should be alert, very anxious, screaming because of the pain in the right lower leg. You are able to follow all verbal and physical commands that the medic gives you.

5 Equipment List

- Live patient, 1
- Manikin, 1
- Stocked M5 bag or CMVS, 1
- SKED/Talon litter, 1

Patient Evaluation Instructor's Information

> **note**
>
> Memorize.

1 Care Under Fire

- All personnel return fire.
- Scene size-up.
- Determines the scene safety.
  - Squad is establishing fire superiority at present.
  - The casualties are not under direct enemy fire at present.
  - Area is secure enough to treat life-threatening injuries prior to movement to the casualty collection point (CCP).
  - Determines the number of patients: 2.
- Rapidly triage casualties.
  - Patient 1: immediate; patient 2: minimal.
  - Directs patient 2 to move to cover, provide assistance as required, move to CCP, and perform self-aid.

> **note** ──────────────────────────────
>
> No further care or evaluation is required for patient 2
> during the trauma scenario; he is only a distraction for
> the medic.

- General impression: Critically injured.
- Airway: Patent.
- Performs immediate treatment: Applies tourniquet.
- Reassures the casualty.
- Requests additional help: Calls for combat lifesaver to assist in moving and providing treatment as required.
- Moves the casualty to a CCP.

2 Tactical Field Care

- Initial assessment, patient 1

> **Vital Signs: Patient 1**
> LOC = Altered mental status
> BP = 70 palpable at carotid
> R = 24 shallow, regular
> P = Weak and thready
> T = Cool

- General impression: Critically injured initially
- C-spine control: Not required
- LOC: Conscious, altered mental status
- Airway: Patent
- Airway adjuncts: Nasopharyngeal airway
- Breathing (opens body armor)
  - Rate increased (anxiety and injury; not airway compromised)
- Circulation
  - Proper blood sweep reveals the following: If tourniquet applied correctly, hemorrhage controlled; other injuries

> **note** ──────────────────────────────
>
> Consider loosening the tourniquet after a dressing and
> bandage has been applied. If bleeding continues,
> retighten the tourniquet.

  - Pulses: Rapid carotid pulse; absent radial pulses bilateral
  - Bleeding: Drying blood to small puncture wounds on right lower leg (not actively bleeding)

- Fluid resuscitation
  - Starts saline lock.
  - Starts IV fluids, 500 mL of Hextend.
  - Re-evaluates after 500 mL of Hextend.
    - The casualty's mental status improves and a palpable radial pulse returns. Do not give additional fluids; maintain saline lock, and observe for changes in vital signs.
  - Covers patient and keeps patient warm.
- Check for additional wounds.
  - Performs a rapid body sweep similar to the blood sweep.
  - Inspects the back.
  - Identifies the right lower leg wounds.
    - Treatment required: Dressing, bandage, and splint

    ### Updated Vital Signs
    LOC = Mental status improving
    BP = 90 palpable at radial
    R = 16 shallow, regular
    P = Regular

- Bandage and splint all wounds.
  - Treatment required: Applies dressing, bandage, and splint to left lower leg.
- Ongoing assessment: Repeated every 5 minutes.
- Packages the patient: Secures to Talon or SKED litter.
- Calls for CASEVAC: Sends a 9-line MEDEVAC request.
- Fills out the FMC (DD1380) and attaches to the patient.
- Administers medications.
  - Pain control: Morphine 5 mg IV every 10 minutes until adequate analgesia is achieved.
  - Antibiotics: Cefotetan 2 g IV push over 3 to 5 minutes, or gatifloxacin 400 mg orally.
- Gathers SAMPLE history prior to administering medications.
  - S = Pain in both legs
  - A = No allergies
  - M = No medications
  - P = No significant past illnesses
  - L = Last meal 3 hours ago
  - E = "I was on patrol and was shot and something exploded pretty close to me."

note

Rapid trauma assessment will be conducted based on mission, enemy, terrain and weather, troops and support available, and time available (METT-T).

3 Critical Measures

o Identifies no immediate threat to casualty or self.
o Applies tourniquet prior to movement to the CCP.
o Identifies signs of shock.
o Establishes saline lock and begins fluid resuscitation with Hextend.
o Applies effective splint.
o Properly packages patient for transport.
o Calls for CASEVAC.

4 Teaching Points

o Apply tourniquet early to significant extremity wounds. Consideration should be given to loosening the tourniquet when the tactical situation allows and after appropriate bandaging and splinting to determine whether bleeding is continuing or the tourniquet can be released.
o If the soldier has no palpable radial pulse and has mental status changes, administer 500 mL Hextend. Then if mental status improves and the radial pulse returns, maintain the saline lock, but do not give additional fluid. If radial pulse does not return or mental status does not improve, administer a second 500 mL of Hextend and re-evaluate.
o Discuss how to administer Narcan if too much morphine is administered and the patient develops respiratory depression.

Scenario 2

1 Scenario History: A loud explosion occurs while soldiers are riding near the tailgate in the back of a cargo Humvee. A 20-year-old rifleman starts to complain of chest pain and shortness of breath. The vehicle has moderate damage and is not able to move. The remainder of the fire team does not appear to have any obvious injuries. The team dismounts and, along with the rest of the squad, is establishing security. The combat lifesaver is calling for the medic.

2 Injuries

o Fragmentary wound to right lower lateral chest
o Tension pneumothorax
o Fragmentary wound, left biceps; minimal bleeding

3 Moulage Instructions

○ Manikin has body armor open.
○ Manikin has one 3-mm puncture wound to the right costal angle midclavicular line. Very minimal bleeding.
○ Left biceps has a 2-cm laceration with a small amount of bleeding.

4 Equipment List

○ Stocked M5 bag or CMVS, 1
○ SKED litter, 1

Patient Evaluation Instructor's Information

> **note**
>
> Memorize.

1 Care Under Fire

○ All personnel establish a secure area.
○ Scene size-up.
  ■ Determines the scene safety.
    • Squad is establishing security at present.
    • No direct enemy fire at present.
    • Area is secure enough to treat life-threatening injuries prior to movement to the CCP.
  ■ Determines the number of patients: 1.
○ Rapidly triage casualty: Immediate, due to progressive severe respiratory distress.
○ Airway: Clear, but respiratory distress noted.
○ Performs immediate treatment.
  ■ None (would be acceptable to consider evaluating the chest followed by decompression with a 14-gauge needle)
○ Reassures the casualty.
○ Requests additional help: Tells the combat lifesaver to assist in moving and providing treatment as required.
○ Moves the casualty to a CCP.

2 Tactical Field Care

○ Initial assessment

Vital Signs
LOC = Alert, anxious
BP = 80 palpable at radial
R = 28, decreased breath sounds (right)
P = Regular
T = Cool

o General impression: Critically injured initially
o C-spine control: Not required
o LOC: Conscious, no altered mental status
o Airway: Patent
o Airway adjuncts: None required
o Breathing (opens body armor)
  ■ Respirations 28 per minute
o Chest
  ■ Anterior: Small puncture wound, right costal angle
    • Treatment required: Decompress the chest with a 14-gauge needle if not done earlier, and apply an occlusive dressing.
  ■ Posterior: No visible injury
o Circulation
  ■ Proper blood sweep reveals the following: Minimal bleeding from the left biceps laceration
    • Treatment required: Dress and bandage.
  ■ Pulses: Radial pulses strong = bilateral
o Fluid resuscitation
  ■ Starts saline lock.
o Check for additional wounds.
  ■ Performs a rapid body sweep similar to the blood sweep.
  ■ Inspects the back.

Updated Vital Signs
LOC = Alert
BP = >90 systolic
R = 20
P = Regular
T = Warm

o Bandage and splint all wounds.
  ■ Applies dressing and bandage to the left arm injury.
o Ongoing assessment: Repeated every 5 minutes.
o Packages the patient.
  ■ Secures to Talon or SKED litter.
  ■ Transports the patient on the injured side.

- Calls for CASEVAC: Sends a 9-line MEDEVAC request.
- Fills out the FMC (DD1380) and attaches to the patient.
- Administers medications.
  - Pain control: Considers the patient's respiratory compromise prior to administering morphine.
  - If morphine is administered, start at low dose (2 mg IV every 10 minutes while monitoring oxygen saturation levels).
  - Antibiotics: Cefotetan 2 g IV push over 3 to 5 minutes, or gatifloxacin 400 mg orally.
- Gathers SAMPLE history prior to administering medications.
  - S = Severe respiratory distress
  - A = No allergies
  - M = No medications
  - P = No significant past illnesses
  - L = Last meal 3 hours ago
  - E = "I was riding in the back of the truck, heard an explosion, and became short of breath, and my left arm got cut and started to bleed."

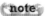

note

Rapid trauma assessment will be conducted based on METT-T.

3 Critical Measures

- Identifies no immediate enemy threat to casualty or self.
- Identifies the early signs and symptoms of a tension pneumothorax and decompresses chest with a 14-gauge needle.
- Applies an occlusive dressing to the chest wound.
- Establishes saline lock.

4 Teaching Points

- Discuss and review pathophysiology associated with tension pneumothorax: why it kills people, and why it needs to be urgently managed.
- All penetrating injuries superior to the umbilicus and inferior to the mandible require an occlusive dressing.

Scenario 3

1 Scenario History: While on patrol in the city of Resith, an infantry platoon starts to receive effective direct small arms fire. A 22-year-old rifleman falls to the ground and begins to scream and hold his left leg. The squad is reacting to contact. Your return fire suppresses the contact. The platoon sergeant tells you, "Work on him for a few minutes, then we have to go."

2 Injuries

o Gunshot wound (GSW) to right thigh with severe bleeding
o Right chest ecchymosis
o Signs and symptoms of shock

3 Moulage Instructions

o Small hole in the manikin's body armor that does not penetrate to the inside
o Right upper quadrant (RUQ) purple ecchymosis over liver due to GSW hitting vest
o GSW entrance: 1-cm entrance wound to right anterior thigh, distal one third
o GSW exit: 5-cm exit wound to the right posterior thigh, proximal one third, with arterial bleeding

4 Equipment List

o Manikin, 1
o Stocked M5 bag or CMVS, 1
o SKED litter, 1

Patient Evaluation Instructor's Information

> **note**
>
> Memorize.

1 Care Under Fire

o All personnel return fire.
o Scene size-up.
  ■ Determines the scene safety.
    • Squad is establishing security at present.
    • The casualty is not under direct enemy fire at present.
  ■ Determines the number of patients: 1.
o Rapidly triage casualty: Immediate, due to the arterial bleeding.
o Airway: Patent (determined by the soldier screaming).
o Performs immediate treatment: Applies tourniquet to right thigh.
o Reassures the casualty.
o Requests additional help: Calls for combat lifesaver to assist in moving and providing treatment as required.
o Moves the casualty to a CCP.

2 Tactical Field Care

o Initial assessment

> **Vital Signs**
> LOC = Altered mental status
> BP = No radial pulses bilateral
> R = 24 per minute
> P = Weak carotid
> T = Cool

o General impression: Critically injured
o C-spine control: Not required
o LOC: Conscious, altered mental status
o Airway: Patent
o Airway adjuncts: Nasopharyngeal airway
o Breathing (opens body armor)
  ■ Respirations 24 per minute
o Chest
  ■ Anterior: RUQ, purple ecchymosis over liver
  ■ Posterior: No visible injury
    • Treatment required: None
o Circulation
  ■ Proper blood sweep reveals the following: If tourniquet was applied correctly, hemorrhage is controlled.

> **note**
> _____
>
> After appropriate fluid resuscitation and bandaging, consider loosening the tourniquet. If bleeding continues, retighten the tourniquet.

  ■ Pulses: Weak, rapid carotid pulse; absent radial pulses bilateral
o Fluid resuscitation
  ■ Starts saline lock.
  ■ Starts IV fluids, 500 mL of Hextend.
  ■ Re-evaluates after 500 mL of Hextend.

> **note**
> _____
>
> If the casualty's mental status improves and a palpable radial pulse returns, hold additional fluids, maintain saline lock, and observe for changes in vital signs.

- Check for additional wounds.
  - Performs a rapid body sweep similar to the blood sweep.
  - Inspects the back.

    Updated Vital Signs
    LOC = Altered mental status
    BP = Systolic BP 60, palpable at carotid
    R = Tachypnea
    P = Weak

- Bandage and splint all wounds.
  - Applies dressing and bandage to previously described injuries.
- Ongoing assessment: Repeated every 5 minutes.
- Packages the patient: Secures to Talon or SKED litter.
- Calls for CASEVAC: Send a 9-line MEDEVAC request.
- Fills out the FMC (DD1380) and attaches to the patient.
- Administers medications.
  - Pain control: Morphine 5 mg IV every 10 minutes until adequate analgesia is achieved.
  - Antibiotics: Cefotetan 2 g IV push over 3 to 5 minutes, or gatifloxacin 400 mg orally.
- Gathers SAMPLE history prior to administering medications.
  - S = Pain to RUQ, right thigh
  - A = No allergies
  - M = No medications
  - P = No significant past illnesses
  - L = Last meal 3 hours ago
  - E = "I was on patrol. We started to receive fire, and I was shot a few times."

    note —————————————————————————

    Rapid trauma assessment will be conducted based on METT-T.

    ————————————————————————————————————

3 Critical Measures

- Identifies no immediate enemy threat to casualty or self.
- Applies tourniquet prior to movement to the CCP.
- Identifies signs of shock.
- Establishes saline lock and begins fluid resuscitation with Hextend.
- Properly packages patient for transport.
- Calls for CASEVAC.

4 Teaching Points

o Apply tourniquet early to significant extremity wounds. Consideration should be given to loosening the tourniquet after appropriate
bandaging and splinting to determine whether bleeding continues or
the tourniquet can be released.

o Administer 500 mL Hextend if the soldier has no palpable radial pulse
and has mental status changes. Then, if mental status improves and
radial pulse returns, hold IV infusion and maintain saline lock. If no
improvement, administer a second 500 mL of Hextend and re-evaluate.

o Discuss how to administer Narcan if too much morphine is administered and patient develops respiratory depression.

Scenario 4

1 Scenario History: While riding in the front of a Humvee through
the city of Resith, your ground assault convoy is hit by an improvised explosive device (IED). The passenger sustains facial
injuries but gets out of the vehicle and attempts to return fire.
The convoy reacts to the attack, establishing fire superiority and
hasty perimeter security. The convoy commander tells you to
get working on the casualty so he can be evacuated and the convoy can get out of this area.

2 Injuries

o Large fragmentary wound to right lower mandible. A large portion
of the bone and tissue is missing.

o Small laceration to right shoulder.

3 Moulage Instructions

o Lower jaw from the right mandibular angle to the middle of the
lower lip is missing. Two teeth are avulsed and attached by a small
ligament. The wound is severely bleeding.

o Right upper deltoid has a small, 4-cm laceration with minimal bleeding.

4 Equipment List

o Manikin, 1

o Stocked M5 bag or CMVS, 1

o SKED litter, 1

Patient Evaluation Instructor's Information

note ————————————————————————

Memorize.

① Care Under Fire

o All personnel return fire.
o Scene size-up.
  ▪ Determines the scene safety.
    • Convoy is establishing security at present.
    • The casualty is not under direct enemy fire at present; no other IEDs have been identified.
  ▪ Determines the number of patients: 1.
o Rapidly triage casualty: Immediate, due to airway compromise and severe bleeding.
o Airway: Patent but threatened.
o Performs immediate treatment.
  ▪ Should be performed in Tactical Field Care phase. If patient is conscious, do you need local anesthesia?
o Reassures the casualty.
o Requests additional help: Calls for combat lifesaver to assist in moving and providing treatment as required.
o Moves the casualty to a CCP.

② Tactical Field Care

o Initial assessment

> **Vital Signs**
> LOC = No altered mental status
> BP = Radial pulses palpable bilateral
> R = 24 per minute
> P = Strong

o General impression: Critically injured.
o C-spine control: Not required.
o LOC: Conscious, no altered mental status.
o Airway: Patent if surgical airway has been administered, pressure dressing applied to facial wounds, and blood cleared from airway.
o Airway adjuncts: Performs a surgical cricothyroidotomy.
o Breathing (opens body armor)
  ▪ Respirations 24 per minute
o Chest: Atraumatic.
o Circulation
  ▪ Proper blood sweep reveals the following:
    • If dressing applied to facial wounds correctly, hemorrhage is controlled
    • Minimal bleeding to laceration on right shoulder
  ▪ Treatment required: Dressing and bandage

- Pulses: Radial pulses present bilateral.
- Fluid resuscitation
  - Starts saline lock.
  - Considers IV fluids.
- Check for additional wounds.
  - Performs a rapid body sweep similar to the blood sweep.
  - Inspects the back.
- Bandage and splint all wounds: Applies dressing and bandage to injuries described previously.

> **Updated Vital Signs**
> LOC = No altered mental status
> BP = Systolic BP at least 90
> R = Tachypnea
> P = Weak
> T = Cool

- Ongoing assessment: Repeated every 5 minutes.
- Packages the patient.
  - Secures to Talon or SKED litter.
  - Transports patient in the prone or recovery position.
- Calls for CASEVAC: Sends a 9-line MEDEVAC request.
- Fills out the FMC (DD1380) and attaches to the patient.
- Administers medications.
  - Pain control: Morphine 5 mg IV every 10 minutes until adequate analgesia is achieved.

note

Considers the patient's airway compromise prior to administering morphine.

  - Antibiotics: Cefotetan 2 g IV push over 3 to 5 minutes, or gatifloxacin 400 mg orally.
- Gathers SAMPLE history prior to administering medications.
  - S = Patient not talking because of facial wounds
  - A = No allergies
  - M = No medications
  - P = No significant past illnesses
  - L = Last meal 3 hours ago
  - E = Unable to get history because of facial wounds

note

Rapid trauma assessment will be conducted based on METT-T.

3 Critical Measures

o Identifies no immediate enemy threat to casualty or self.
o Identifies immediate threat to patient's airway.
o Performs a surgical cricothyroidotomy.
o Applies dressing to facial wounds.
o Establishes saline lock.
o Properly packages patient for transport.
o Calls for CASEVAC.

4 Teaching Points

o Perform a surgical cricothyroidotomy because of massive facial trauma. The only way to effectually treat facial bleeding is to pack the mouth, which cannot be done until the airway is secured.

Scenario 5

1 Scenario History: While riding in the back of a Humvee transporting unleaded gas to a nongovernmental organization, you hear a loud explosion. The lead vehicle has hit an IED and a large flash (fire) is seen. The vehicle has rolled over. Small flames are coming from the back of the vehicle. The driver and TC were able to get out of the vehicle and are moving to the cover of the other vehicles. The two personnel in the back have been thrown from the vehicle and are lying a few feet away. Both have sustained injuries. The convoy commander is establishing security and tells you to start working on the casualties.

2 Injuries

o Patient 1
  ▪ Facial burns with developing facial edema and shortness of breath
  ▪ Decreased level of consciousness
  ▪ Fractured right lower tibia; pulses intact
  ▪ Dislocated right shoulder
o Patient 2
  ▪ Fragmentary wounds to both lower legs
  ▪ Second degree burn to left arm

3 Moulage Instructions

o Patient 1
  ▪ Manikin has burns to face; mustache and nasal hairs have been burnt.
  ▪ Second degree burns of approximately 5% body surface area.

- Right lower leg mid-shaft tibia has a simple fracture with ecchymosis.
- Right shoulder deformity from dislocation.

o Patient 2
- Small tears in BDU pants. Nomex gloves on both hands with evidence of fire damage.
- Eight to ten 1- to 2-mm puncture wounds to right lower leg, with minimal bleeding.
- Second degree burn on left arm anterior from elbow to wrist.

④ Patient 2 Instructions

o You should be alert, very anxious, screaming because of the pain from your burn and fragmentary wounds. You are able to follow all verbal and physical commands that the medic gives you. No further history will be given, except stating that you will be OK and that treatment should be given to patient 1.

⑤ Equipment List

o Live patient, 1
o Manikin, 1
o Stocked M5 bag or CMVS, 1
o SKED litter, 1

Patient Evaluation Instructor's Information

> **note**
>
> Memorize.

① Care Under Fire

o All personnel return fire and establish security.
o Scene size-up.
- Determines the scene safety.
  - Convoy personnel are establishing fire superiority and security at present.
  - The casualties and all personnel attempting to provide care are in danger from the fire and gasoline that was in the back of the vehicle.
  - The area is not secure enough to treat life-threatening injuries prior to movement to the CCP.
- Determines the number of patients: 2.
o Rapidly triage casualties.
- Patient 1, immediate; patient 2, minimal.

- Directs patient 2 to help move casualty 1 to a secure area by grabbing the casualty's vest and dragging the casualty to cover.
- While under cover, direct patient 2 to perform self-care.

> **note**
>
> No further care or evaluation is required for patient 2 during the trauma scenario; he is only a distraction for the medic.

o Performs immediate treatment: No treatment until away from the vehicle and secure.
o Reassures the casualty.
o Requests additional help: Calls for combat lifesaver to assist in moving and providing treatment as required.
o Moves the casualty to a CCP.

2 Tactical Field Care

o Initial assessment, patient 1

> **Vital Signs: Patient 1**
> LOC = Altered mental status
> BP = All pulses palpable bilateral
> R = 42 per minute
> P = Strong bilateral
> T = Warm

o General impression: Critically injured
o C-spine control: Required
o LOC: Altered mental status
o Airway: Compromised due to developing facial edema and burns
o Airway adjuncts: Surgical cricothyroidotomy
o Breathing (opens body armor): Rate decreasing after a surgical cricothyroidotomy
o Circulation
 ■ Proper blood sweep reveals: No life-threatening hemorrhage
  · Patient grimaced with movement of right leg and shoulder.
o Pulses: Rapid pulses = bilateral upper and lower extremities
o Bleeding: No active bleeding
o Fluid resuscitation
 ■ Starts saline lock.
 ■ Starts IV fluids (Ringer's lactate, normal saline)

Use the following burn formula, or give a fluid bolus of 500-1000 cc. Formula: Take the percentage of body area burned, multiplied by the patient's weight in kilograms, then multiply that by 4 cc of fluid. Administer 50% of the total fluids over 8 hours.

Updated Vital Signs

LOC = Altered mental status
BP = All pulses palpable bilateral
R = 30 per minute
P = Strong bilateral
T = Warm

- Check for additional wounds.
  - Performs a rapid body sweep similar to the blood sweep. Inspects the back also.
  - Identifies the right lower leg wounds.
- Bandage and splint all wounds.
  - Applies anatomical splint to right lower leg.
  - Applies burn dressings to face and head.
  - Applies sling and swath to right arm.
- Packages the patient and calls for CASEVAC.
- Fills out the FMC (DD1380) and attaches it to the patient.
- Administers medications.
  - Pain control: Morphine 5 mg IV every 10 minutes until adequate analgesia is achieved.
  - Considers possible airway compromise prior to administering analgesics.
  - Antibiotics: Cefotetan 2 g IV push over 3 to 5 minutes.
- Gathers SAMPLE history prior to administering medications.
  - S = Unable to gather information from patient
  - A = No allergies (determined by checking identification tags)
  - M = No medications
  - P = No significant past illnesses (assumption due to active duty soldier)
  - L = Last meal: unknown
  - E = Patient not able to talk because of respiratory distress

Rapid trauma assessment will be conducted based on METT-T.

(3) Critical Measures

o Identifies immediate threat to casualty and self.
o Moves to the CCP or safe area before rendering care.
o Identifies airway compromise and treats with airway adjunct.
o Establishes saline lock and administers IV fluids.

(4) Teaching Points

o Discuss what airway adjuncts can be used to maintain the airway with facial and tongue edema above the vocal cords.
o Supraglottic airway adjuncts are not recommended for inhalation-type injuries. The type of airway used must be distal to the vocal cords, or the localized edema will occlude it.
o Discuss C-spine control when patient's life is endangered.

Scenario 6

(1) Scenario History: While on patrol in the city of Resith, an infantry platoon starts to receive effective machine gun fire. A 30-year-old platoon sergeant falls to the ground and begins to hold his groin area and scream in pain. The platoon is reacting to contact. Your return fire suppresses the contact. The platoon leader tells you to take care of the platoon sergeant.

(2) Injuries

o Multiple gunshot wounds (GSWs) to the pelvis and groin area with severe bleeding
o Fractured pelvis

(3) Moulage Instructions

o Manikin has three 1- to 2-cm GSWs to right posterior buttocks with a large exit wound in the anterior right inguinal region with severe bleeding.

(4) Equipment List

o Manikin, 1
o Stocked M5 bag or CMVS, 1
o SKED litter, 1

Patient Evaluation Instructor's Information

note

Memorize.

1 Care Under Fire

o All personnel establish a secure area.
o Scene size-up.
  ■ Determines the scene safety.
    · Platoon is establishing security at present.
    · No effective enemy fire at present.
    · Area is not secure enough to treat life-threatening injuries prior to movement to the CCP.
    · Moves casualty behind cover to begin lifesaving care.
  ■ Determines the number of patients: 1.
o Rapidly triage casualty: Immediate, due to massive bleeding.
o Airway: Patent.
o Reassures the casualty.
o Requests additional help: Calls for combat lifesaver to assist in moving and providing treatment as required.
o Moves the casualty to a CCP.

2 Tactical Field Care

o Initial assessment

> **Vital Signs**
> LOC = Altered
> BP = Unknown, systolic BP <80
> R = 28 rapid, shallow
> P = Rapid carotid
> T = Cool

o General impression: Critically injured
o C-spine control: Not required
o LOC: Altered mental status
o Airway: Patent
o Airway adjuncts: Nasopharyngeal airway
o Breathing (opens body armor)
  ■ Respirations 18 per minute
o Chest: No visible injury
o Circulation
  ■ Proper blood sweep reveals the following: Severe arterial bleeding from right inguinal exit wound
  ■ Treatment required
    · Applies dressing and bandage to groin (packing of groin wound).
    · Applies dressing and bandage to wounds on buttocks.
    · Uses poncho or poncho liner under buttocks, twists tails to stabilize pelvis.

○ Pulses: Radial pulses absent
○ Fluid resuscitation
  ■ Starts saline lock.
  ■ Starts IV fluids, 500 mL of Hextend.
  ■ Re-evaluates after 500 mL of Hextend.
  ■ Administers second 500 mL of Hextend.

> **note**
>
> If the casualty's mental status improves and a palpable radial pulse returns, hold additional fluids, maintain saline lock, and observe for changes in vital signs.

  Updated Vital Signs
  LOC = Altered
  BP = Palpable carotid
  R = 24
  P = Weak, thready radial
  T = Cool

○ Check for additional wounds.
  ■ Performs a rapid body sweep similar to the blood sweep.
  ■ Inspects the back.
○ Bandage and splint all wounds.
  ■ Applies dressing and bandage to injuries discussed previously.
○ Ongoing assessment: Repeated every 5 minutes.
○ Packages the patient.
  ■ Secures to Talon or SKED litter.
○ Calls for CASEVAC: Sends a 9-line MEDEVAC request.
○ Fills out the FMC (DD1380) and attaches to the patient.
○ Administers medications.
  ■ Pain control: Morphine 5 mg IV every 10 minutes until adequate analgesia is achieved.
  ■ Antibiotics: Cefotetan 2 g IV push over 3 to 5 minutes, or gatifloxacin 400 mg orally.
○ Gathers SAMPLE history prior to administering medications.
  ■ S = Pain in groin and hips
  ■ A = No allergies
  ■ M = No medications
  ■ P = No significant past illnesses
  ■ L = Last meal 3 hours ago .
  ■ E = Not able to give accurate information

Rapid trauma assessment will be conducted based on METT-T.

3 Critical Measures

o Identifies possible immediate enemy threat to casualty or self.
o Identifies life-threatening bleeding and packs groin wound.
o Identifies and stabilizes fractured pelvis.
o Establishes saline lock/IV and administers Hextend.

4 Teaching Points

o Discuss methods to stop bleeding in groin and axillary regions.
o Discuss and review the pathophysiology, early and late signs, and symptoms of shock.
o Discuss and review fluid resuscitation.
o Discuss treating a fractured pelvis using a sheet, blanket, or poncho liner.
o Discuss how to get a patient with a fractured pelvis on a Talon litter since logrolling is not recommended for pelvic fractures.
o Discuss sliding the patient onto a SKED litter.

Scenario 7

1 Scenario History: While sitting in the open hatch of a Bradley fighting vehicle (BFV), the TC removes his helmet and is taking a break. A loud explosion is heard behind the hatch, and the hatch door falls onto his head, which slams the TC's head between the hatch and vehicle. The TC is rendered unconscious. Another BFV crewmember saw the insurgent throw an explosive device and killed him by direct fire. Other members in the vehicle call for the medic. Due to METT-T, it takes approximately 1 hour for the medic to arrive. By the time the medic arrives, the casualty is out of the vehicle and sitting on the ground talking. A buddy stated that he applied a dressing to his head wound and that the casualty has vomited a few times.

2 Injuries

o Depression with laceration over the left parietal region of the skull

3 Moulage Instructions

o 6-cm depression on left side of head
o 10-cm scalp laceration over depression

4 Equipment List

o Manikin, 1
o Stocked M5 bag or CMVS, 1
o SKED/Talon litter, 1

Patient Evaluation Instructor's Information

> **note**
>
> Memorize.

1 Care Under Fire

o All personnel establish security. Area is secure by the time the medic arrives.
o Scene size-up.
  ■ Determines the scene safety.
    • Squad has established security.
    • The casualty is not under direct enemy fire at present.
    • Area is secure enough to treat life-threatening injuries prior to movement to the CCP.
  ■ Determines the number of patients: 1.
o Rapidly triage casualties: Immediate.
o General impression: Critically injured.
o Airway: Patent.
o Performs immediate treatment: Stabilizes the patient's head.
o Reassures the casualty.
o Requests additional help: Calls for combat lifesaver to assist in providing treatment as required.
o Moves the casualty to a CCP: Designates the vehicle as the CCP.

2 Tactical Field Care

o Initial assessment

Vital Signs
LOC = Alert
BP = 160/90
R = 12
P = 50
T = Warm

o General impression: Critically injured
o C-spine control: Required

- LOC: Conscious at first, developing altered mental status, followed by unconsciousness while the medic is evaluating the patient
- Airway: Patent, followed by threatened as Glasgow Coma Scale rating drops to below 8
- Airway adjuncts
  - Initial: Nasopharyngeal airway with altered level of consciousness
  - Advanced: Combitube when the patient becomes unconscious
- Breathing: Rate decreased
- Circulation
  - Proper blood sweep reveals the following: Laceration of scalp. No brain or gray matter seen.
  - Pulses: Bradycardia.
- Bleeding
  - 10-cm laceration to scalp. Blood is coming through the original dressing.
  - Applies or reinforces the dressing to scalp.
- Fluid resuscitation
  - Starts saline lock.
  - Covers patient and keeps warm.

  ### Updated Vital Signs
  LOC = Unconscious
  BP = 210/150
  R = 10
  P = 45

- Check for additional wounds.
  - Performs a rapid body sweep similar to the blood sweep.
  - Inspects the back.
- Bandage and splint all wounds.
  - Treatment required: Applies dressing and bandage to the head wound.
- Ongoing assessment: Repeated every 5 minutes.
- Packages the patient.
  - States that he will secure the patient to a long spineboard and place on a Talon or SKED litter when the equipment arrives.
  - Elevates the head of litter.
  - Prepares suction device to handle emesis as required.
- Calls for CASEVAC: Sends a 9-line MEDEVAC request (requests a spineboard).
- Fills out the FMC (DD1380) and attaches to the patient.
- Administers medications.
  - Pain control: Not required due to condition.
  - Antibiotics: Cefotetan 2 g IV push over 3 to 5 minutes.

o Gathers SAMPLE history prior to administering medications.
  ■ S = Headache, neck pain, cut on head
  ■ A = No allergies
  ■ M = No medications
  ■ P = No significant past illnesses
  ■ L = Last meal 3 hours ago
  ■ E = "I was taking a break when I heard a noise and got hit in the head with something."

> **note**
>
> Rapid trauma assessment will be conducted based on METT-T.

3 Critical Measures

o Identifies no immediate threat to casualty or self.
o Applies cervical collar.
o Identifies signs of head injuries.
o Establishes appropriate airway.
o Establishes saline lock but does not begin fluid resuscitation.
o Properly packages patient for transport.
o Calls for CASEVAC.

4 Teaching Points

o Assume a cervical spine injury by the mechanism of injury.
o An altered level of consciousness is the hallmark of brain injury.
o The Cushing response to elevated intracranial pressure consists of hypertension, bradycardia, and a decreased respiratory rate. The hypertension represents the brain's effort to maintain cerebral perfusion pressure.
o Never assume that the brain injury is the cause of hypotension.
o Classic epidural hematoma scenario is a head injury followed by loss of consciousness, followed by a lucid interval, followed by coma and then a fixed and dilated pupil on the side of the lesion.

Scenario 8

1 Scenario History: While on patrol in the city of Resith, an infantry squad starts to receive direct small arms fire followed by a loud explosion. A 19-year-old rifleman falls to the ground and begins to scream about pain in both arms and hold his right hand, which is partially severed. The injured soldier is calling for the medic.

2 Injuries

- Partial amputation to the right hand just below the wrist
- Multiple fragmentary wounds to both upper extremities

3 Moulage Instructions

- Right hand partial amputation just below the wrist with arterial bleeding.
- Both upper extremities have ten to fifteen 1- to 2-mm puncture wounds with small amount of bleeding.

4 Equipment List

- Live patient, 1
- Manikin, 1
- Stocked M5 bag or CMVS, 1
- SKED/Talon litter, 1

Patient Evaluation Instructor's Information

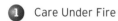

note

Memorize.

1 Care Under Fire

- All personnel return fire.
- Scene size-up.
  - Determines the scene safety.
    - Squad is establishing fire superiority at present.
    - The casualties are not under direct enemy fire at present.
    - Area is secure enough to treat life-threatening injuries prior to movement to the CCP.
  - Determines the number of patients: 1.
- Rapidly triage casualties: Immediate.
- General impression: Critically injured.
- Airway: Patent.
- Performs immediate treatment: Applies tourniquet.
- Reassures the casualty.
- Requests additional help: Calls for combat lifesaver to assist in moving and providing treatment as required.
- Moves the casualty to a CCP.

2 Tactical Field Care

- Initial assessment

Vital Signs
LOC = Altered mental status
BP = 70 palpable at carotid
R = 24 shallow, regular
P = Weak and thready
T = Cool

o General impression: Critically injured initially
o C-spine control: Not required
o LOC: Conscious, altered mental status
o Airway: Patent
o Airway adjuncts: Nasopharyngeal airway
o Breathing (opens body armor)
  ■ Rate increased (anxiety and injury, not airway compromise)
o Circulation
  ■ Proper blood sweep reveals the following: If tourniquet applied
    correctly, hemorrhage is controlled; other injuries

---

note

Consider loosening the tourniquet after a dressing and
bandage has been applied. If bleeding continues,
retighten the tourniquet.

---

o Pulses: Rapid carotid pulse, absent radial pulses bilateral
o Bleeding: Drying blood in small puncture wounds to left lower leg
  (not actively bleeding)
o Fluid resuscitation
  ■ Starts saline lock.
  ■ Starts IV fluids, 500 mL of Hextend.
  ■ Re-evaluates after 500 mL of Hextend.
    • The casualty's mental status improves and a palpable radial
      pulse returns. Do not give additional fluids, maintain saline lock,
      and observe for changes in vital signs.
  ■ Covers patient and keeps warm.

      Updated Vital Signs
      LOC = Mental status improving
      BP = 90 palpable at radial
      R = 16 shallow, regular
      P = Regular

o Check for additional wounds.
  ■ Performs a rapid body sweep similar to the blood sweep.
  ■ Inspects the back.

- Identifies the right and left arm wounds.
- Treatment required: Dressing, bandage, and splint.
○ Bandage and splint all wounds.
  - Treatment required
    • Applies dressing, bandage, splint, and sling to right hand and wrist.
    • Applies dressing, bandage to left arm.
○ Ongoing assessment: Repeated every 5 minutes.
○ Packages the patient: Secures to Talon or SKED litter.
○ Calls for CASEVAC: Sends a 9-line MEDEVAC request.
○ Fills out the FMC (DD1380) and attaches to the patient.
○ Administers medications.
  - Pain control: Morphine 5 mg IV every 10 minutes until adequate analgesia is achieved.
  - Antibiotics: Cefotetan 2 g IV push over 3 to 5 minutes, or gati-floxacin 400 mg orally.
○ Gathers SAMPLE history prior to administering medications.
  - S = Pain in both arms
  - A = No allergies
  - M = No medications
  - P = No significant past illnesses
  - L = Last meal 3 hours ago
  - E = "I was on patrol and was shot and something exploded pretty close to me."

> **note**
>
> Rapid trauma assessment will be conducted based on METT-T.

③ Critical Measures

○ Identifies no immediate threat to casualty or self.
○ Applies tourniquet prior to movement to the CCP.
○ Identifies signs of shock.
○ Establishes saline lock and begins fluid resuscitation with Hextend.
○ Applies effective splint.
○ Properly packages patient for transport.
○ Calls for CASEVAC.

④ Teaching Points

○ Apply tourniquet early to significant extremity wounds. Consideration should be given to loosening the tourniquet when the tactical situation allows and after appropriate bandaging and splinting to determine whether bleeding continues or the tourniquet can be released.

o If the soldier has no palpable radial pulse and his mental status changes, administer 500 mL Hextend. Then if mental status improves and radial pulse returns, maintain saline lock, but do not give additional fluid. If radial pulse does not return or mental status does not improve, administer a second 500 mL of Hextend and re-evaluate.
o Discuss how to administer Narcan if too much morphine is administered and patient develops respiratory depression.

Scenario 9

1 Scenario History: While on patrol in the city of Resith, an infantry platoon starts to receive effective machine gun fire. A 30-year-old platoon sergeant falls to the ground and begins to hold his axillary region and scream of pain. The platoon is reacting to contact. Your return fire suppresses the contact. The platoon leader tells you to take care of the platoon sergeant.

2 Injuries
o GSW to the right upper back and axillary region with severe bleeding
o Pneumothorax

3 Moulage Instructions
o Manikin has two 1- to 2-cm GSWs to right posterior upper back, with a large exit wound in the right axillary region with severe bleeding.

4 Equipment List
o Manikin, 1
o Stocked M5 bag or CMVS, 1
o SKED litter, 1

Patient Evaluation Instructor's Information

> **note** ————————————————————————
>
> Memorize.
>
> ————————————————————————————————

1 Care Under Fire
o All personnel establish a secure area.
o Scene size-up.
  ■ Determines the scene safety.
    • Platoon is establishing security at present.
    • No effective enemy fire at present.

- Area is not secure enough to treat life-threatening injuries prior to movement to the CCP.
- Moves casualty behind cover to begin lifesaving care.
  - Determines the number of patients: 1.
- Rapidly triage casualty.
  - Immediate, due to severe respiratory distress
  - Immediate, due to massive bleeding
- Airway: Clear, but respiratory distress noted.
- Reassures the casualty.
- Requests additional help: Calls for combat lifesaver to assist in moving and providing treatment as required.
- Moves the casualty to a CCP.

2 Tactical Field Care

- Initial assessment

  ### Vital Signs
  LOC = Altered
  BP = Unknown, systolic BP <80
  R = 28 rapid, shallow
  P = Rapid carotid
  T = Cool

- General impression: Critically injured
- C-spine control: Not required
- LOC: Conscious, altered mental status
- Airway: Patent
- Airway adjuncts: Nasopharyngeal airway
- Breathing (opens body armor)
  - Respirations 28 per minute
- Chest
  - Anterior: No visible injury
  - Posterior: GSW to right upper back
    - Treatment required: Apply both an occlusive and pressure dressing.
- Circulation
  - Proper blood sweep reveals the following: Severe arterial bleeding from right axillary exit wound
  - Treatment required
    - Dressing and bandage to axillary (packing of axillary wound)
    - Occlusive dressing
  - Pulses: Radial pulses absent
- Fluid resuscitation
  - Starts saline lock.
  - Starts IV fluids, 500 mL of Hextend.

- Re-evaluates after 500 mL of Hextend.
- Administers second 500 mL of Hextend.

> **note**
>
> If the casualty's mental status improves and a palpable radial pulse returns, hold additional fluids, maintain saline lock, and observe for changes in vital signs.

Updated Vital Signs
LOC = Altered
BP = Palpable carotid
R = Progressive respiratory distress
P = Weak and thready, radial

o Check for additional wounds.
   - Performs a rapid body sweep similar to the blood sweep.
   - Inspects the back, if not completely done earlier.
o Bandage and splint all wounds.
   - Applies dressing, bandage to injuries described earlier.
o Ongoing assessment: Repeated every 5 minutes.
o Progressive respiratory distress occurs after application of occlusive dressings.
   - Treatment required: Decompress the chest with a 14-gauge needle.
o Packages the patient: Secures to Talon or SKED litter.
o Calls for CASEVAC: Sends a 9-line MEDEVAC request.
o Fills out the FMC (DD1380) and attaches to the patient.
o Administers medications.

> **note**
>
> Consider respiratory compromise and symptoms of shock before administering medications.

   - Pain control: Morphine 5 mg IV every 10 minutes until adequate analgesia is achieved.
   - Antibiotics: Cefotetan 2 g IV push over 3 to 5 minutes.
o Gathers SAMPLE history prior to administering medications.
   - S = Pain in back and armpit
   - A = No allergies
   - M = No medications
   - P = No significant past illnesses
   - L = Last meal 3 hours ago
   - E = Not able to give accurate information

Rapid trauma assessment will be conducted based on METT-T.

---

③ Critical Measures

o Identifies possible immediate enemy threat to casualty or self.
o Identifies life-threatening bleeding and packs axillary wound.
o Establishes saline lock/IV and administers Hextend.
o Identifies the early signs and symptoms of a tension pneumothorax and decompresses chest with a 14-gauge needle.
o Applies an occlusive dressing to the chest wound.

④ Teaching Points

o Discuss methods to stop bleeding in groin and axillary regions.
o Discuss and review the pathophysiology, early and late signs, and symptoms of shock.
o Discuss and review pathophysiology associated with tension pneumothorax, including why it kills people and why it needs to be urgently managed.
o All penetrating injuries superior to the umbilicus and inferior to the mandible require an occlusive dressing.
o Discuss and review fluid resuscitation.

Scenario 10

① Scenario History: While on patrol in the city of Resith, an infantry platoon starts to receive effective direct small arms fire. A 22-year-old rifleman falls to the ground and begins to scream of pain in his back. The platoon is reacting to contact. Your return fire suppresses the contact. The platoon sergeant tells you, "Work on him for a few minutes, then we have to go."

② Injuries

o Gunshot wound (GSW) to right costal vertebral angle, with minimal bleeding (kidney injury)
o Signs and symptoms of shock

③ Moulage Instructions

o Small hole in body armor that penetrates to the inside.
o GSW entrance: 1-cm entrance wound to right costal vertebral angle; no exit wound.

④ Equipment List

o Manikin, 1
o Stocked M5 bag or CMVS, 1
o SKED litter, 1

Patient Evaluation Instructor's Information

> **note** ——————————————————————
>
> Memorize.

① Care Under Fire

o All personnel return fire.
o Scene size-up.
  ■ Determines the scene safety.
    • Squad is establishing security at present.
    • The casualty is under direct enemy fire at present.
  ■ Determines the number of patients: 1.
o Rapidly triage casualty: Immediate, due to GSW in back.
o Airway: Patent (determined by the soldier screaming).
o Performs immediate treatment: None.
o Reassures the casualty.
  ■ Tells the casualty to remain still as if he were dead.
  ■ Tells the casualty he will come get him when the direct fire is suppressed.
o Requests additional help: Calls for combat lifesaver to assist in moving and providing treatment as required.
o Moves the casualty to a CCP.
  ■ Enemy fire is suppressed. The medic and combat lifesaver grab the casualty and drag him to the CCP.

② Tactical Field Care

o Initial assessment

> **Vital Signs**
> LOC = Altered mental status
> BP = No radial pulses bilateral
> R = 24 per minute
> P = Weak carotid
> T = Cool

o General impression: Critically injured
o C-spine control: Not required

- LOC: Conscious, altered mental status
- Airway: Patent
- Airway adjuncts
  - Initial: Nasopharyngeal airway.
  - Later: After patient becomes unconscious, use Combitube.
- Breathing: Respirations 24 per minute
- Chest
  - Anterior: No visible injury
  - Posterior: No visible injury
  - Treatment required: None
- Back
  - 2-cm GSW to right costal vertebral angle with minimal bleeding
  - Treatment required: Dressing and bandage
- Circulation
  - Proper blood sweep reveals the following: No other injuries
  - Pulses: Weak, rapid carotid pulse; absent radial pulses bilateral

    ### Updated Vital Signs
    LOC = Altered mental status
    BP = Systolic BP 60 palpable at carotid
    R = Tachypnea
    P = Weak

- Fluid resuscitation
  - Starts saline lock.
  - Starts IV fluids, 500 mL of Hextend.
  - Re-evaluates after 500 mL of Hextend.
  - Administers additional 500 mL of Hextend.

    note

    If the casualty's mental status improves and a palpable radial pulse returns, hold additional fluids, maintain saline lock, and observe for changes in vital signs.

- Check for additional wounds.
  - Performs a rapid body sweep similar to the blood sweep.
  - Inspects the back if not done earlier.

    ### Updated Vital Signs
    LOC = Unconscious
    BP = Systolic BP 50
    R = Tachypnea
    P = Unable to palpate
    T = Cool, clammy

o Bandage and splint all wounds.
o Ongoing assessment: Repeated every 5 minutes.
o Packages the patient.
  ■ Secures to Talon or SKED litter.
o Calls for CASEVAC: Sends a 9-line MEDEVAC request.
o Fills out the FMC (DD1380) and attaches to the patient.
o Administers medications.

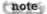

> Considers respiratory compromise and symptoms of
> shock before administering medications.

  ■ Pain control: Morphine 5 mg IV every 10 minutes until adequate
    analgesia is achieved.
  ■ Antibiotics: Cefotetan 2 g IV push over 3 to 5 minutes.
o Gathers SAMPLE history prior to administering medications.
  ■ S = Pain to right mid back
  ■ A = No allergies
  ■ M = No medications
  ■ P = No significant past illnesses
  ■ L = Last meal 3 hours ago
  ■ E = "I was on patrol. We started to receive fire and I was shot."

> Rapid trauma assessment will be conducted based on
> METT-T.

3 Critical Measures

o Identifies immediate enemy threat to casualty and self.
o Identifies signs of shock.
o Establishes saline lock and begins fluid resuscitation with Hextend.

4 Teaching Points

o Administer 500 mL Hextend if the soldier has no palpable radial
  pulse and his mental status changes. Then if mental status improves
  and radial pulse returns, hold IV infusion and maintain saline lock. If
  no improvement is made, administer a second 500 mL of Hextend
  and re-evaluate.
o Patients with massive internal injuries can die even when all the
  treatment is appropriate and done in a timely manner.

Algorithms

Anaphylactic Shock Management

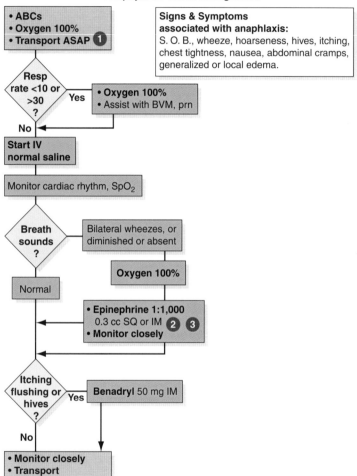

Signs & Symptoms associated with anaphlaxis:
S. O. B., wheeze, hoarseness, hives, itching, chest tightness, nausea, abdominal cramps, generalized or local edema.

- ABCs
- Oxygen 100%
- Transport ASAP ❶

Resp rate <10 or >30 ? — **Yes** →
- Oxygen 100%
- Assist with BVM, prn

No

Start IV normal saline

Monitor cardiac rhythm, SpO₂

Breath sounds ? → Bilateral wheezes, or diminished or absent

Oxygen 100%

Normal

- Epinephrine 1:1,000 0.3 cc SQ or IM ❷ ❸
- Monitor closely

Itching flushing or hives ? — **Yes** → Benadryl 50 mg IM

No

- Monitor closely
- Transport

1 **Bee sting:** gently remove stinger if still present.
2 **Two (2) dilutions of epinephrine are available:** 1:1,000 is appropriate for SQ, IM, or SL injections, <u>1:10,000 is for IV or ET use ONLY.</u> Be sure to give the appropriate dilution.
3 **Contact Medical Control** if symptoms/signs persist.

Burn Management

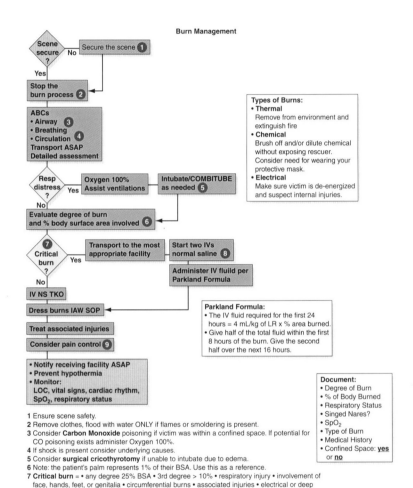

1 Ensure scene safety.
2 Remove clothes, flood with water ONLY if flames or smoldering is present.
3 Consider **Carbon Monoxide** poisoning if victim was within a confined space. If potential for CO poisoning exists administer Oxygen 100%.
4 If shock is present consider underlying causes.
5 Consider **surgical cricothyrotomy** if unable to intubate due to edema.
6 Note: the patient's palm represents 1% of their BSA. Use this as a reference.
7 **Critical burn** = • any degree 25% BSA • 3rd degree > 10% • respiratory injury • involvement of face, hands, feet, or genitalia • circumferential burns • associated injuries • electrical or deep chemical burns • underlying medical history • age < 10 or > 50 years.
8 Start IVs within unburned areas if possible. Burned areas may be used if needed.
9 **Morphine** 5-10 mg IV (adult).

Chest Tube Insertion

- ABCs
- Oxygen 100%
- Assist ventilations, prn
- Transport ASAP

Select site: affected side, 2nd intercostal space, (nipple level) anterior to the midaxillary line.

Cleanse site with povidone.

Locally anesthetize the skin and rib periosteum.

Make a 2-3 cm horizontal incision at the predetermined site and bluntly dissect through the subcutaneous tissues just over the top of the 6th rib.

Puncture the parietal pleura with the tip of the clamp and spread the tissues.

With the index finger of the nondominant hand, trace the clamp into the incision to avoid injury to other organs and clear any adhesions or clots.

With the index finger of the nondominant hand remaining in place, clamp the proximal end of the chest tube and insert into the chest cavity to the desired length.

Look for "fogging" of the chest tube with expiration.

Connect the end of the chest tube to the Heimlich valve.

Suture the tube in place.

Apply dressings: wrap tube with petrolatum gauze then cut 4 x 4's. Tape the tube to the chest.

Monitor SpO$_2$, cardiac rhythm, and clinical status

Items Needed:
9" Peans
1-0 Armed Suture
Povidone Solution
No. 10 Scalpel
No. 36-38 Chest Tube
Heimlich Valve
4x4's
Petrolatum Gauze
18-Gauge Needle
10-cc Syringe
1% Lidocaine
Chux
2" Tape
Sterile Gloves

Document:
- Airway
- Respiratory Status
- SpO$_2$
- Vital Signs
- Cardiac Rhythm
- Lung Sounds Before and After Chest Tube Insertion
- Skin Color
- Chest Rise/Excursion
- Capillary Refill
- Response to Treatment
- Site Selection

Combitube SA

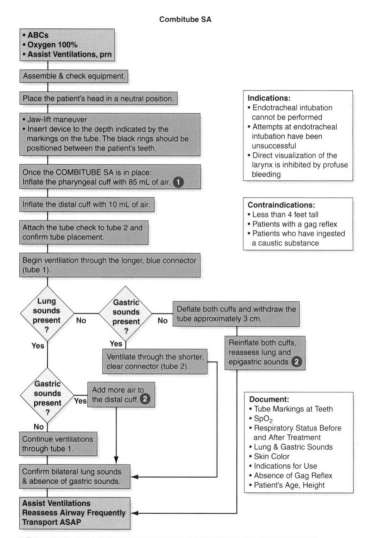

- ABCs
- Oxygen 100%
- Assist Ventilations, prn

Assemble & check equipment.

Place the patient's head in a neutral position.

- Jaw-lift maneuver
- Insert device to the depth indicated by the markings on the tube. The black rings should be positioned between the patient's teeth.

Once the COMBITUBE SA is in place: Inflate the pharyngeal cuff with 85 mL of air. ❶

Inflate the distal cuff with 10 mL of air.

Attach the tube check to tube 2 and confirm tube placement.

Begin ventilation through the longer, blue connector (tube 1).

Lung sounds present? — No → **Gastric sounds present?** — No → Deflate both cuffs and withdraw the tube approximately 3 cm.

↓ Yes .... ↓ Yes

Reinflate both cuffs, reassess lung and epigastric sounds ❷

Ventilate through the shorter, clear connector (tube 2).

Gastric sounds present? — Yes → Add more air to the distal cuff. ❷

↓ No

Continue ventilations through tube 1.

Confirm bilateral lung sounds & absence of gastric sounds.

Assist Ventilations Reassess Airway Frequently Transport ASAP

Indications:
- Endotracheal intubation cannot be performed
- Attempts at endotracheal intubation have been unsuccessful
- Direct visualization of the larynx is inhibited by profuse bleeding

Contraindications:
- Less than 4 feet tall
- Patients with a gag reflex
- Patients who have ingested a caustic substance

Document:
- Tube Markings at Teeth
- SpO$_2$
- Respiratory Status Before and After Treatment
- Lung & Gastric Sounds
- Skin Color
- Indications for Use
- Absence of Gag Reflex
- Patient's Age, Height

1 This seals the device in the posterior pharynx behind the hard palate. More air may be added to the pharyngeal cuff if an inadequate seal is detected during ventilation.

2 At no time should the patient's airway or ventilatory status be compromised. If placement is unsuccessful, remove the device and return to naso/oropharyngeal airway and assist ventilations via bag-valve-mask.

3 When using a tube check with a Combitube you are confirming that the tube is in the esophagus (tube check should not re-inflate).

NOTE: This protocol is ONLY to be used with the Combitube SA and does NOT apply to the STANDARD Comitube.

Needle Decompression

• ABCs
• Oxygen 100%
• Assist ventilations, prn
• Transport ASAP

Select site: affected side, 2nd intercostal space, mid-clavicular line.

Items Needed:
• 10-14 gauge 2.5-3.0 needle with catheter
• Povidone swab

Cleanse site with povidone.

Remove the Luer-Lok from the distal end of the catheter, insert the needle/cath over the rib into the intercostal space and puncture the parietal pleura.

Remove the needle from the catheter and listen for a sudden escape of air.

Leave catheter in place, converting the tension to an open pneumothorax.

Ensure tension has been relieved. If not, repeat procedure.

Auscultate breath sounds FREQUENTLY and monitor PT status.

Document:
• Airway
• Respiratory Status
• SpO_2
• Vital Signs
• Cardiac Rhythm
• Lung Sounds Before and After Decompression
• Skin Color
• Chest Rise/Excursion
• Capillary Refill
• Response to Treatment
• Site Selection

Monitor SpO_2, cardiac rhythm, and clinical status

Signs & Symptoms to look for when assessing tension pneumothorax
• <u>Increases respiratory distress</u>
• <u>Unilateral chest movement</u>
• Decreased breath sounds on the affected side
• Distended neck veins
• Tracheal deviation
• Shock

Orotracheal Intubation

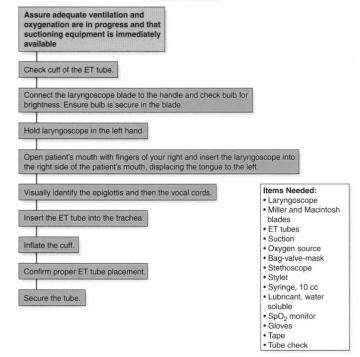

Assure adequate ventilation and oxygenation are in progress and that suctioning equipment is immediately available

Check cuff of the ET tube.

Connect the laryngoscope blade to the handle and check bulb for brightness. Ensure bulb is secure in the blade.

Hold laryngoscope in the left hand.

Open patient's mouth with fingers of your right and insert the laryngoscope into the right side of the patient's mouth, displacing the tongue to the left.

Visually identify the epiglottis and then the vocal cords.

Insert the ET tube into the trachea.

Inflate the cuff.

Confirm proper ET tube placement.

Secure the tube.

Items Needed:
- Laryngoscope
- Miller and Macintosh blades
- ET tubes
- Suction
- Oxygen source
- Bag-valve-mask
- Stethoscope
- Stylet
- Syringe, 10 cc
- Lubricant, water soluble
- SpO$_2$ monitor
- Gloves
- Tape
- Tube check

Document:
- ABCs
- Detailed Assessment
- Vital Signs
- SpO$_2$, ETCO$_2$
- Glasgow Coma Scale
- Tube Check Results
- Lung Sounds
- Absence of Epigastric Sounds
- Skin Color
- Teeth to ET Tube Tip Depth
- Communication with Medical Control

1 Maintain strict c-spine precautions if potential for c-spine injury exists.
2 Avoid applying pressure on teeth or lips.
3 Never use a prying motion.
4 Advance the ET tube: ensure the tube cuff is 1 to 2.5 cm below the vocal cords (on a adult).
5 Anytime the patient goes **30 seconds without ventilation,** stop the procedure and hyperventilate for 30-60 seconds before procedure is re-attempted.
6 Intubation is <u>only to be attempted twice</u>. After two unsuccessful attempts are made, transition to the COMBITUBE.

F.A.S.T. 1

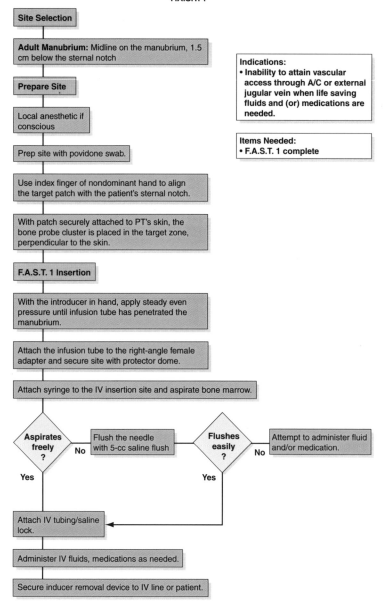

Site Selection

Adult Manubrium: Midline on the manubrium, 1.5 cm below the sternal notch

Prepare Site

Local anesthetic if conscious

Prep site with povidone swab.

Use index finger of nondominant hand to align the target patch with the patient's sternal notch.

With patch securely attached to PT's skin, the bone probe cluster is placed in the target zone, perpendicular to the skin.

F.A.S.T. 1 Insertion

With the introducer in hand, apply steady even pressure until infusion tube has penetrated the manubrium.

Attach the infusion tube to the right-angle female adapter and secure site with protector dome.

Attach syringe to the IV insertion site and aspirate bone marrow.

Aspirates freely ? — No → Flush the needle with 5-cc saline flush → **Flushes easily ?** — No → Attempt to administer fluid and/or medication.

Yes ↓   Yes ↓

Attach IV tubing/saline lock.

Administer IV fluids, medications as needed.

Secure inducer removal device to IV line or patient.

Indications:
• Inability to attain vascular access through A/C or external jugular vein when life saving fluids and (or) medications are needed.

Items Needed:
• F.A.S.T. 1 complete

Surgical Cricothyroidotomy

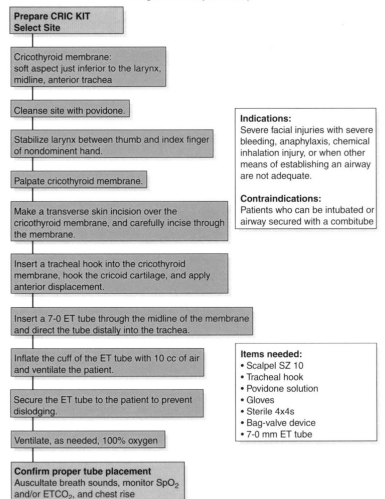

Prepare CRIC KIT
Select Site

Cricothyroid membrane:
soft aspect just inferior to the larynx,
midline, anterior trachea

Cleanse site with povidone.

Stabilize larynx between thumb and index finger
of nondominent hand.

Palpate cricothyroid membrane.

Make a transverse skin incision over the
cricothyroid membrane, and carefully incise through
the membrane.

Insert a tracheal hook into the cricothyroid
membrane, hook the cricoid cartilage, and apply
anterior displacement.

Insert a 7-0 ET tube through the midline of the membrane
and direct the tube distally into the trachea.

Inflate the cuff of the ET tube with 10 cc of air
and ventilate the patient.

Secure the ET tube to the patient to prevent
dislodging.

Ventilate, as needed, 100% oxygen

Confirm proper tube placement
Auscultate breath sounds, monitor SpO_2
and/or $ETCO_2$, and chest rise

Indications:
Severe facial injuries with severe
bleeding, anaphylaxis, chemical
inhalation injury, or when other
means of establishing an airway
are not adequate.

Contraindications:
Patients who can be intubated or
airway secured with a combitube

Items needed:
• Scalpel SZ 10
• Tracheal hook
• Povidone solution
• Gloves
• Sterile 4x4s
• Bag-valve device
• 7-0 mm ET tube

Line 1. Location of pickup site (grid or latitude/longitude)	**1.**
Line 2. Frequency and callsign at pickup site	**2.**
Line 3. Number of patients by precedence	**3.**
a. Urgent-nonsurgical (i.e., heat, disease, etc.)—evacuate within 2 hours	A.
b. Urgent-surgical (all trauma)—need immediate surgical care to stabilize	B.
c. Priority—evacuate within 4 hours	C.
d. Routine—evacuate within 24 hours	D.
e. Convenience—evacuate when possible	E.
Line 4. Special equipment required	**4.**
A—None	A.
B—Hoist	B.
C—Extraction equipment	C.
D—Ventilator	D.
Line 5. Number of patients by type:	**5.**
L + # of litter patients	L.
A + # of ambulatory patients	A.
Line 6. WARTIME: Security of pickup site	**6.**
N—No enemy troops	
P—Possible enemy troops in the area	
E—Confirmed enemy troops in area (use caution)	
X—Currently engaged with enemy troops (armed escort recommended)	
Line 7. MARKING OF PICKUP SITE	**7.**
A—VS 17 panel	A.
B—Pyro, type	B.
C—Smoke, color	C.
D—None	D.
E—Other	E.
Line 8. Patient nationality and status (if known)	**8.**
A = US/Coalition Military, Nationality =	A.
B = US/Coalition Force Civilian, Nationality =	B.

C = Non-coalition Force Soldier, Nationality =	C.
D = Non-US/Coalition Force Soldier, Nationality =	D.
E = Enemy prisoner of war	E.
F = High value target (armed escort required)	F.
Line 9. WARTIME: NBC contamination (N = nuclear/B = biological/ C = chemical)	**9.**

US Medevac Units Operating in Area

Unit:	Unit:
Loc./Proximity:	Loc./Proximity:
HF:	HF:
FM:	FM:
DNVT:	DNVT:
Callsign:	Callsign:
Iridium Phone:	Iridium Phone:
Unit:	Unit:
Loc./Proximity:	Loc./Proximity:
HF:	HF:
FM:	FM:
DNVT:	DNVT:
Callsign:	Callsign:
Iridium Phone:	Iridium Phone:

Backup Contacts for Ground Evac

If you cannot contact the nearest BCT TOC or Medevac team/unit you may contact the following HQ command TOC's with a 9-Line Medevac request:

Unit:	Unit:
Loc./Proximity:	Loc./Proximity:
HF:	HF:
FM:	FM:
DNVT:	DNVT:
Callsign:	Callsign:
Iridium Phone:	Iridium Phone:

International Humanitarian Law and the Geneva Conventions

Customary international law and lawmaking treaties such as the Geneva and Hague Conventions regulate the conduct of hostilities on land. The rights and duties set forth in the conventions are part of the supreme law of the land. The United States is obligated to adhere to these conventions even when an opponent does not. Department of Defense (DOD) and Army policies require that we conduct operations in a manner consistent with these obligations.

During all military operations, members of the U.S. armed forces must be prepared to detain personnel who are no longer willing or able to continue fighting, and other personnel based on detention criteria (threat to U.S. forces, threat to members of the local population, and other security interests). For the medical community, this also means to be prepared to take into custody, protect, and medically care for all categories of potential detainees.

International humanitarian law (IHL) is the body of rules which, in wartime, protects people who are not or are no longer participating in the hostilities. Its central purpose is to limit and prevent human suffering in times of armed conflict.

The Geneva Conventions are a series of treaties signed by most nations of the world. The first convention, signed in 1864, established rules that protect soldiers who are wounded to the extent that they can no longer serve as a combatant. The original rules, or conventions, were expanded over the years and by 1949 included provisions for the protection of: wounded and sick members of the armed forces on land and sea, shipwrecked members of armed forces, medical personnel, medical facilities and equipment, wounded and sick support personnel accompanying the armed forces, military chaplains, civilians who spontaneously take up arms to repel an invasion, hospital ships, prisoners of war (POWs)/enemy prisoners of war (EPWs), and civilians. The conventions and their protocols specifically protect people who do not take part in the fighting (civilians, medics, chaplains, humanitarian workers, and other civilians who are providing humanitarian assistance) and those who can no longer fight (wounded or sick troops and POWs/EPWs).

Under the laws of war, certain persons are protected as "noncombatants," including:

○ Civilians: Civilians and civilian property may not be the subject of a military attack. Civilians are people who are not members of the enemy's armed forces and do not take part in the hostilities. Journalists and members of the International Committee of the Red Cross (ICRC) are also given protection as "civilians."

○ Wounded and sick in the field and at sea: Soldiers who have fallen by reason of sickness or wounds and who cease to fight are to be respected and protected.

○ Prisoners of war: Surrender may be made by any means that communicates the intent to give up. There is no clear-cut rule as to what constitutes surrender. However, most agree that surrender constitutes a cessation of resistance and placement of one's self at the direction of the captor. Captors must respect (not attack) and protect (care for) those who surrender.

○ Chaplains: Chaplains are considered protected persons.

○ Medical personnel: Medical personnel are specifically identified in the 1st Geneva Convention. "Medical personnel exclusively engaged in the search for, or the collection, transport, or treatment of the wounded and the sick . . . shall be respected and protected in all circumstances." This includes permanent medical personnel (doctors, nurses, physician assistants, medics) and support personnel.

Medical personnel receive two forms of protection under the Geneva Conventions: protection from attack and protection upon capture.

○ Protection from attack: The Geneva Convention protects medical personnel because they are noncombatants. Medical personnel who perform non-medical duties harmful to the enemy lose their protective status.

○ Protection upon capture: If captured, medical personnel are considered "retained personnel," not POWs. Retained personnel:
   ■ Can only be required to perform medical duties.
   ■ Must receive at least all the benefits conferred on POWs.
   ■ May be retained only as long as needed to tend to prisoners of war who are sick and wounded.
   ■ Must be returned when "retention is not indispensable."
   ■ Must obey POW camp rules.

Treating and Guarding Detainees

Detainee Classification

The DOD definition of the word "detainee" refers to any person captured or otherwise detained by an armed force. As a matter of policy, all detainees will be treated in accordance with the principles applicable to enemy prisoners of war unless and until a more precise legal status is determined.

There are four categories of detainees listed under the Geneva Conventions. These persons are entitled to the privileges of the Geneva Conventions:

○ Enemy Prisoner of War (EPW) is defined as a detained person as described in the Geneva Conventions. In particular, one who, while engaged in combat under orders of his or her government, is captured by the armed forces of the enemy.
○ Civilian Internee (CI) is an individual interned during an international armed conflict for security reasons, for protection, or because they have committed an offense (insurgent, criminal) against the detaining power.
○ Retained Persons (RP) are enemy personnel who are either medical personnel, chaplains, or are in voluntary aid societies (Red Cross, etc.). They are eligible to be considered retained personnel.
○ Other Detainee (OD) is a person in the custody of U.S. armed forces who has not yet been classified as an EPW, CI, or RP.

In reference to the Global War on Terror (GWOT), there is an additional classification of detainees who, through their own conduct, are not entitled to the privileges and protection of the Geneva Conventions. These personnel are classified as enemy combatants (EC). These people are still entitled to be treated humanely.

Care and Treatment of Detainees

Our nation's law requires that we afford certain rights to people captured on the battlefield. They are basic rights, but every disciplined soldier needs to be aware of them. Affording these protections is also of military value. We also comply with these rules because it helps us on the battlefield. If the enemy knows we will treat him with dignity and respect, he is more likely to surrender. We also hope that these rights will be afforded to our soldiers if they should become prisoners of war.

Always initially treat a captured person as an EPW. Process them according to the "Five Ss":

○ Search them: Immediately search them for weapons, ammunition, equipment, and documents with intelligence value. EPW/RP will be allowed to retain personal effects of sentimental or religious value.
○ Segregate them: Place them into groups of enlisted, noncommissioned officers, and officers. Individuals presumed to have intelligence value should be separated immediately from other EPWs.

○ Silence them: Segregation should prevent prisoners from communicating with each other by voice or visual means.

○ Safeguard them: While they are your prisoner, you are responsible for their safety.

○ Speed them to the rear: The wounded EPW patient is evacuated to the rear as soon as their medical condition permits. Then:
  ■ Tag them.

You can fulfill your military mission and still treat these people in a humane manner. Many of these people will be victims of war, and some may be enemy soldiers, but once captured, they are entitled to the same humane treatment.

The medical standard of care for detainees is the same as for U.S. forces, in accordance with the Geneva Conventions, "Members of the armed forces . . . who are wounded or sick shall be respected and protected in all circumstances." They must be treated humanely, be cared for without adverse distinction founded on sex, race, nationality, religion, or similar criteria, and attempts on their lives shall be strictly prohibited. The conventions further require that detainees will not be left without medical assistance and care.

Priority for medical treatment shall be based on the severity of the wound/injury. The most urgent wounded/sick soldiers will be treated first, regardless of the uniform they are wearing.

Initial Actions upon Capture

1 Noninjured detainees will be humanely evacuated from the combat zone and into appropriate channels as quickly as possible. Sick and wounded detainees will be evacuated separately, but in the same manner as U.S. and allied forces.

2 Body cavity exams or searches may be performed for valid medical reasons with the verbal consent of the patient. However, these exams should not be performed as part of a routine intake physical examination. Body cavity searches are to be conducted only when there is a reasonable belief that the detainee is concealing an item that presents a security risk.

3 If possible, a body cavity exam will be conducted by personnel of the same gender.

Evacuation and Care of Detainees

Those units designated to hold and evacuate detainees will categorize sick and wounded detainees in their custody as walking or nonwalking (litter) wounded. These personnel will be delivered to the nearest medical facility (MTF) and evacuated through medical channels.

Detainees will only be transferred to another MTF if medically stable to do so and will never be transferred out of country without Secretary of Defense (SECDEF) approval.

Providing Medical Care Required for Persons in Confinement

- In-Processing Medical Requirements:
  - All detainees will receive a screening medical examination during in-processing. This examination will include a medical history and physical examination, a screening chest x-ray, dental screening, mental health screening, and height and weight measurement. As previously discussed, it will not include a body cavity search unless medically indicated.
  - This physical screening exam is conducted to detect lice, communicable diseases (TB, STDs), and to assess overall health, nutritional, and hygiene status.
  - A medical record will be created during in-processing and all screening information will be recorded in it. Medical records will accompany detainees throughout the medical system and a copy will be provided to the detainee upon release, if requested.
  - Each facility shall provide copies of the applicable Geneva Conventions for detainees in their own language.
- Outpatient Care
  - Sick call for detainees requiring medical attention will be held daily. EPW/RP/CI will *not* be denied medical care. To the extent possible, detainees will be cared for separately from Coalition Forces and civilians. Every effort should be made to have female health care providers screen and care for female detainees. MTF staff, to include security personnel, will maintain a professional appearance and military bearing at all times while working with detainees. Medical support to EPW, RP, CI, and other detainees includes:
  - First aid and all sanitary aspects of food service.
  - Preventive medicine.
  - Professional medical services and medical supply.
  - Coordinating the use of medically trained EPW, CI, RP personnel, and medical material.

- The United States is bound to take all sanitary measures necessary to ensure clean and healthy camps to prevent epidemics. Every camp will have an infirmary. Any detainee with a contagious disease, mental condition, or other illness as determined by the medical officer will be isolated from the other patients.
- Detainees will be immunized against other diseases as recommended by the Theater Surgeon.
- Detainees suffering from serious diseases or whose condition necessitates special treatment, surgery, or hospital care must be admitted to any military or civilian medical unit where treatment can be given. Special facilities will be available for the care and the rehabilitation of the disabled. Detainee evacuation outside the theater of operations requires SECDEF approval.
- The detaining authorities shall, upon request, issue to every detainee who has undergone treatment, an official certificate indicating the nature of the injury/illness and the duration and type of treatment received. A duplicate certificate will be sent to the ICRC. The detaining authority will ensure medical personnel complete the appropriate medical records: SF 88 (Report of Medical Examination), SF 600 (Chronological Record of Medical Care), and DA Form 3444 (Treatment Record). Documentation of medical care will occur at every level of medical care and be transported with the detainee.
  - Medical inspections will be held at least once a month, where each detainee will be weighed and the height recorded. The purpose of these inspections will be to monitor the general state of health, nutrition, and cleanliness of prisoners and to detect contagious diseases (TB, STDs, HIV, lice).
  - Camp commanders will conduct periodic and detailed sanitary inspections. Detainees will be provided with sanitary supplies, service, and facilities necessary for their personal cleanliness and sanitation. Separate latrine facilities will be provided for each gender.
- Detainees will not be handcuffed or tied, except to ensure safe custody or when prescribed by a responsible medical officer as needed to control a medical case requiring restraint.
- The inhumane treatment of detainees is prohibited and not justified by the stress of combat or deep provocation. At no time will detainee medical information be available for interrogation purposes. Medical personnel must, however, report any information obtained during the course of medical care which could affect the safety and security of other detainees or Coalition Forces.

- Detainees will be protected against all acts of violence to include rape, forced prostitution, assault, theft, and bodily injury. They will not be subjected to medical or scientific experiments.
- During transport, detainees will have sufficient food and drinking water to keep them in good health, and will be provided adequate clothing, shelter, and medical attention.
- Personnel resources to guard detainee medical patients are provided by the Echelon Commander; medical personnel do not guard detainee patients.

Training Scenario

You are a recent graduate of the 91W Combat Medic Course and you have been assigned to a medical platoon in a forward support company. Your unit is scheduled to deploy to Iraq. Your platoon sergeant informed that your duties will consist of providing care to enemy detainees in a confinement facility. As you reflect on your training in the 91W Course you have many questions:

1 What kind of human rights are commonly violated in an armed conflict?

Armed conflict can result in a violation of a wide range of legal rules. There are restrictions on who can be targeted. Only combatants in opposing forces and military objects can be targeted. Very often woman and children suffer disproportionately, and will be specifically targeted for abuse and attack. Sometimes, members of groups are targeted on racial, religious, or ethnic grounds and this is also prohibited.

2 Do support personnel who do not directly treat patients have a protected status?

Those who look after the administration of medical units and establishments are similarly protected, as they are an integral part of the medical service of the military, which could not function without them.

3 In order to maintain their protected status can medical personnel do *anything* other than treat patients?

Yes. The rule is that they may not perform acts that are harmful to the enemy, as this will jeopardize their protected status. They can do various administrative-type duties that do not harm the enemy.

4 What if medical personnel are assigned to guard a nonmedical facility?

This will jeopardize their protective status. They should not be assigned to administrative duties not directly connected with the operation/administration of the medical unit.

5 Could a commander order the removal of the red cross emblem from a vehicle and still use the vehicle for a medical purpose?

Yes, there is no requirement to affix a red cross to anything. This however, may jeopardize the protection it would be entitled to, as the enemy may not recognize it.

6 In order to enhance operations security (OPSEC), can the red cross emblem be camouflaged (e.g., use a dark brown cross with a light sand-color background)?

To be protected under the Geneva Conventions, the emblem must be red on a white background.

7 Suppose a commander wants to use an ambulance for a non-medical purpose (i.e., transport combat troops). Can he do so?

Yes, but he must cover up the red cross or other protective emblem; however, this will result in the ambulance becoming a legitimate target.

8 What about the opposite situation, can I take a combat vehicle and put a red cross emblem on it so it will not be attacked while it is performing a nonmedical function?

No. Misuse of the medical emblem in this manner is a war crime.

9 What happens if medical personnel use defensive weapons to fire at enemy soldiers?

If you start acting as combatants, the enemy will respond accordingly. So long as the enemy is complying with the Law of War, medical personnel may not use weapons in an offensive mode. It is only when the enemy violates the Law of War that medical personnel may use these defensive weapons in combat, otherwise you will lose your protected status.

10 What if medical personnel are carrying grenades and have machine guns?

It would be hard to argue that these weapons are defensive, and this could jeopardize the protection of the medical establishment.

11 Why should we care about the welfare of the enemy?

After the 1991 Gulf War, many Iraqi prisoners were reluctant to leave, and asked to remain in our POW facilities. Think of all of the lives that were saved when thousands of Iraqi soldiers gave up. Which would you rather have, 10,000 enemy soldiers surrendering or 10,000 enemy soldiers wanting to shoot you? If the enemy thinks we will kill them if they surrender, then why would they surrender? We want to encourage the enemy to surrender, so we do not want enemy prisoners dying in our custody.

12 Suppose wounded and hungry enemy soldiers are under your medical care. You think they know the locations of enemy units in the area. Can you deny them medical treatment or food until they provide that information to interrogators?

No. The Geneva Convention that protects EPWs prohibits forcing a prisoner into giving information of any kind, whatsoever.

13 Your unit is conducting a search in a built-up area. As they go from building to building, a few weapons are discovered. But in one home, they find some interesting art objects and decide to take them. Would this be a crime?

Yes, taking the objects is a violation of the Law of War. They have no right to the property. If during the same search, they deliberately smash dishes or burn books and clothing, they would also be violating the Law of War by destroying property when it is militarily unnecessary.

Patient Notes

DATE_____ TIME_____

PATIENT NAME_____

SSN_____UNIT_____

SEX_____ AGE_____ HT_____ WT_____

CHIEF COMPLAINT_____

_____

_____

_____

_____

_____

LOC_____ TEMP._____ PULSE_____ BP_____

RESPIRATIONS_____ PUPILS_____

LUNG SOUNDS_____

OTHER PERTINENT FINDINGS_____

_____

_____

_____

MEDICATIONS_____

_____

ALLERGIES_____

MEDICAL HISTORY_____

_____

_____

Notes

Notes